Karina Fanelli

Cochlear Implant Programming

Karina Fanelli

Cochlear Implant Programming

Audiological management of technological
resources to optimize auditory performance

ScienciaScripts

Imprint

Any brand names and product names mentioned in this book are subject to trademark, brand or patent protection and are trademarks or registered trademarks of their respective holders. The use of brand names, product names, common names, trade names, product descriptions etc. even without a particular marking in this work is in no way to be construed to mean that such names may be regarded as unrestricted in respect of trademark and brand protection legislation and could thus be used by anyone.

Cover image: www.ingimage.com

This book is a translation from the original published under ISBN 978-613-9-41017-0.

Publisher:
Sciencia Scripts
is a trademark of
Dodo Books Indian Ocean Ltd. and OmniScriptum S.R.L publishing group

120 High Road, East Finchley, London, N2 9ED, United Kingdom
Str. Armeneasca 28/1, office 1, Chisinau MD-2012, Republic of Moldova, Europe
Printed at: see last page
ISBN: 978-620-6-52157-0

INDEX

DEDICATED

To my parents, for being the best model of effort, perseverance, humility, empathy, generosity and honesty.

To my family and friends who supported this initiative.

To my teachers, in order of appearance, Lic. Claudia Kac, Lic. Alejandra Moyano, Lic. Susana Erdocian, Dr. Manuel Manrique, Dr. Alicia Huarte, MA Norma Pallares, Prof. Vicente Diamante for being the solid and generous guides who knew how to lead my professional training.

To my bosses, MA Norma Pallares and Prof. Vicente Diamante who knew how to instill in me practices of scientific and human quality and gave me a space to perform my work.

To my classmates, Lic. Marcela Wolman. Celia Braun Acosta, MA Norma Pallares and TAV Marcela Garrido, and to the students of Therapeutic audiology, who daily motivate me to improve the level of teaching.

INTRODUCTION

The cochlear implant is a hearing aid device that currently provides consistent information between 188 to 7938 Hz to people with severe or profound hearing loss without age limit.

The selection of candidates for cochlear implants is generally governed by the 2000 FDA marketing approval that considers:

For adults:

- Older than +18 years with tonal thresholds >50 to 90dB HL Bilateral

- With pre-peri- or post-lingual hearing loss

- Performance <50% in the worst and 60% in the best of recognition Sentences in recorded lists

For children:

- Between 12 to 24m:

- Tonal thresholds >90dB bilateral HL

- Between 2 to 17 a:

- Tonal thresholds >70dB bilateral HL

- With 3-6 m of use Headphones

o IT-Mais and speech perception test for small children

o Older: <30% recognition MLNT/LNT

Due to the lack of updated criteria for the indication of cochlear implants, as in other countries, in Argentina, leading otologists in the field met to outline a consensus on the new criteria for cochlear implants based on technological advances and the best auditory performance achieved. (http://faso.org.ar/imagenes/informe.pdf)

These modifications in the criteria allowed access to cochlear implants to many patients with limited benefits with the use of hearing aids and improved their performance and quality of life.

We cannot fail to mention the beginnings of commercialization in Argentina in 1987. Both audiologists and doctors and auditory rehabilitators had to incorporate new practices and strategies to their daily work in order to provide patients with better possibilities to access speech. This is how Norma Pallares, together with Graciela Brick and Monica Matti, performed the first cochlear implant calibration in Buenos Aires that year. From then on, with their generous contributions on the management of severe and profound hearing loss, different professionals dedicated a great part of their work to the diffusion of the benefits and the optimization of the practices to obtain the greatest benefit with the use of the device.

The audiological management for the programming of cochlear implants requires, in addition to a full knowledge of the internal and external components, functioning, measurements and electrical stimulation parameters to be modified in order to provide the patient with consistent access to speech, the management of evaluation protocols and post cochlear implant follow-up to monitor and supervise the evolution of auditory and language skills. We must keep in mind that our audiological work conditions the future not only of the patient but also of the family and social environment.

CURRENT COCHLEAR COCHLEAR IMPLANT SYSTEM COMPONENTS [R]

o ***External component***

Consisting of the speech processor. We currently have a behind-the-ear model and a cordless out-of-ear model for those with pinna discomfort or aesthetic requirements. All have wireless connectivity and allow access to telephone, TV, remote speech/noise and multimedia content with great efficiency and ease.

As for the processor model, from an audiological point of view, it is suggested to opt for the behind-the-ear model in the first instance. However, if the patient is a spectacle wearer, has a small or soft pinna or if he/she refers pain in any support site, if he/she perspires excessively, if he/she is a spectacle wearer or has important esthetic needs, the out-of-ear processor is recommended. Some patients who have refused cochlear implant placement for years now agree to surgery because they have this type of wireless processor.

As far as performance and hearing quality are concerned, the latest model is always superior, and consequently it is the one we suggest to purchase. There are limitations of social coverage, so sometimes the indication is changed for a current but cheaper device.

The devices marketed in Argentina are:

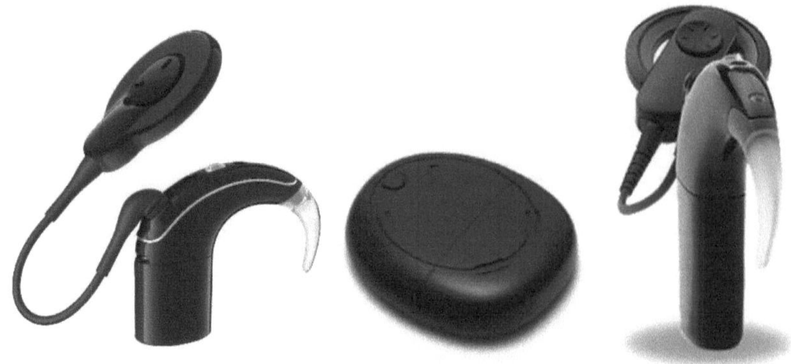

<table>
<tr><td>Nucleus Behind-The-Ear Speech Processor[R] 7 -
  CP1000</td><td>Nucleus Out-of-Hearing Speech Processor[R] Kanso - CP950</td><td>Nucleus Behind-The-Ear Speech Processor[R] 6 - CP910</td></tr>
</table>

(Images courtesy of Cochlear [R])

All feature dual microphone technology, automatic signal processing, Bluetooth connectivity, IP57 resistance and accessories for children, sports and water.

The life span of the device is estimated between 4 to 5 years, which may vary according to use, care, handling, perspiration, ambient humidity and physical activity. Therefore, the physical condition and the hearing quality of the processor should be monitored audiologically at each control in order to be able to consider its upgrade in a timely manner. In Argentina, the processors have a 3-year warranty, after which a repair or a complete upgrade of the external equipment may be requested. The audiologist should be able to evaluate which is the most convenient situation depending on the state of the rest of the external components (batteries, chargers, cable, coil) and the technology.

o *Internal component*

An implantable device, surgically placed, that receives the encoded signal from the external processor and delivers an electrical signal to the ganglion cells of the auditory nerve.

There are different models, straight and perimodiolar, all with 22 intracochlear electrodes and 2 reference electrodes that make it possible to establish a circulation circuit for the electrical charge delivered.

The choice of the device and the ear to be implanted is in the hands of the Otologist, who will make this decision based on the audiological studies, the state of the inner ear, the patient's hearing experience and the previous use of hearing aids. It is therefore essential to record these data in the clinical history and perform the audiological studies in a thorough manner. The validity of the studies for the indication is one month considering the high incidence of progressive hearing loss.

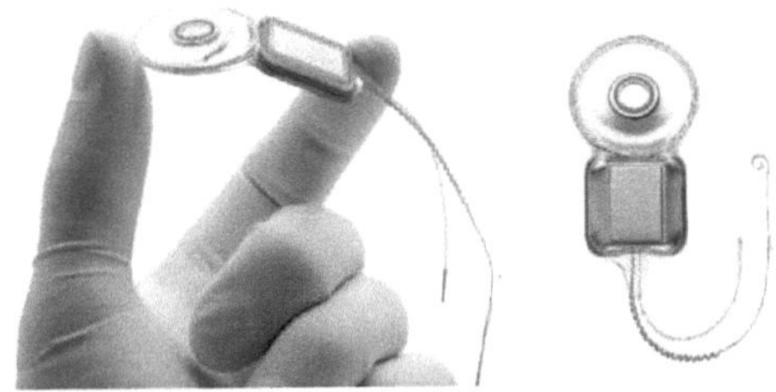

CI512 Implant (Images courtesy of Cochlear)[R]

This internal component is checked at each programming. If changes in its condition are detected, it should be referred to an otologist for evaluation by means of imaging and physical examination.

DESCRIPTION OF THE CURRENT COCHLEAR COCHLEAR IMPLANT SYSTEM PROGRAMMING PARAMETERS[R] THAT MAKE UP A MAP

As for Cochlear devices[R] , the Custom Sound software has a combination of basic stimulation parameters, by which programming is initiated. But it also has a wide range of advanced tools to modify the characteristics of the standard electrical stimulation when the patient does not respond according to the expectations for the case.

This combination of electrical stimulation parameters will form a programming MAP (MAP: measurable auditory percept) with which the cochlear implant will be put into operation.

As a didactic approach, as Wolfe and Schafer(I) do in their book, we will describe the different parameters by groups, according to the effect generated in the electrical stimulation.

Parameters affecting the time-coded signal

o **_Stimulation mode_**

The stimulation mode determines the location of the indifferent electrode in relation to the active electrode (2). It indicates **_how_** the channels are connected to form an electrical circuit through which the electrical current delivered to the auditory nerve is mobilized (1). They can be modified channel by channel through the data grid on the screen or on all channels from the MAP Parameters control or by creating a map and selecting a different mode there. (2) See graph 1.

Depending on where the reference electrode is located (indifferent, ground or return electrode), the stimulation mode can be:

■ Monopolar (MP): consisting of an intacocochlear electrode and an extracochlear electrode that serves as a return electrode. All current implants use this stimulation mode by default (1). In MP1 mode, the active electrode uses the ball electrode as reference, in MP2 the reference electrode is located in the internal receiver/stimulator and MP1+2 when the active electrode is related to the two extracochlear electrodes as reference (MPI and MP2). The latter is used by default in the Nucleus24 models.

■   Bipolar: it is a mode used with Nucleus22 models in which both electrodes -active and reference- are intacoclear, because the system does not have extracoclear electrodes. The active electrode is next to the reference electrode (BP) and can be separated by 1 place BP+1 or 2 places BP+2 and so on (1).

■   Comon ground: is a mode used for diagnosis and not for stimulation. In this mode one intracochlear electrode is active and the rest of the intracochlear electrodes act as reference (1).

Although the BP stimulation mode provides the most focused stimulation, the MP stimulation allows to provide a tonotopic signal through the cochlea, requiring lower current level and therefore longer battery life. Moreover, the stimulation pattern is gradual allowing interpolation of stimulation levels (1). Therefore, the choice of the stimulation mode is kept by default in MP1+2, except in special cases, where we must modify it due to failure of MP1 or MP2 or due to deterioration of the auditory performance, we try with a BP mode.

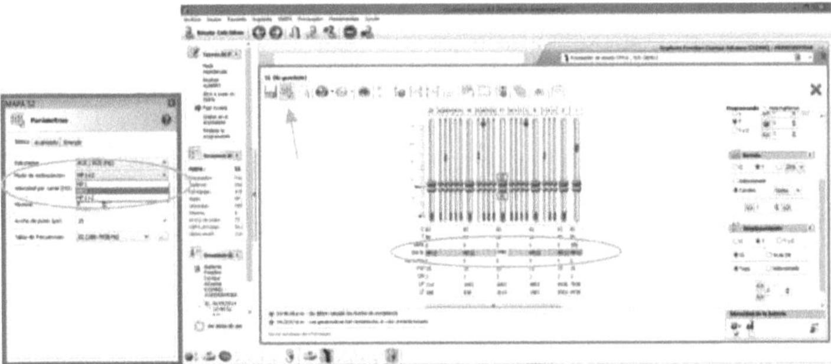

Figure 1: Choice of stimulation mode.

- ○ **Coding Strategies**

The sound coding strategy defines how the speech processor analyzes the acoustic signals and **what it** encodes to send to the auditory nerve ganglion cells via the internal component.

The coding of the acoustic signal through the cochlear implant is based on three principles:

- *Tone* : the incoming signal is divided into frequency bands through filter banks that will be represented by independent channels ranging from 188 to 7938Hz (2).

- *Place or Tonotopy*: This information divided into frequency bands will be carried through the channel to each electrode that will stimulate a specific area of the cochlea. The apical electrodes will transmit low frequency bands and the basal electrodes high frequencies, respecting the cochlea tonotopic organization (3), which still does not correspond to the normal one. The frequency band of the implants is lower and the place where the electrode stimulates does not coincide in frequency.

- *Velocity*: The coded signal will be applied with a certain *periodicity* on the ganglion cells of the auditory nerve, which have a certain conductive capacity that is restricted from 1000Hz (3). Each otological history determines a characteristic of electrical behavior of the first neuron of the 8th pair. Therefore, it is important to contemplate the performance and verify which is the speed that provides the greatest benefit.

The various coding or signal processing strategies developed for multichannel cochlear implants differ in how they extract speech information and how they present it to the electrode. They can be divided into:

- *Waveform-based strategies*: they represent the waveform in a pulsatile way, filtering the speech in frequency bands. In the Nucleus cochlear implant, the CIS (Continuous Sequential Sampling) strategy is available: it is created at the Reaserch Triangle Institute, in order to solve the interaction and overlapping of the electrodes using successive, not simultaneous, biphasic pulses. In this way, one electrode is stimulated at a time and the amplitude is given by the extraction of the wave envelope. It uses non-linear compression to ensure output within the patient's electrical dynamic range. This strategy was a precursor of later strategies (3).

When the input signal arrives at the processor it is sent to a filter bank and divided into discrete frequency bands. The tonotopic organization is preserved by the signal processing and represented by the electrodes placed on the cochlea. All chosen electrodes are stimulated sequentially during each stimulation circle with the amplitude corresponding to the energy of each channel (1).

This strategy stimulates the same channel during each stimulation cycle despite spectral changes of the information. It divides the acoustic information in bands from 188-7938 Hz between 4 to 12 channels (3).

The stimulation rate per channel has a directly proportional effect on speech recognition. This can be varied manually as well as the pulse width. According to different studies, some patients benefit from 833 pulses/s, others from 1365 and others from 2525 pulses/s (3).

Currently, we have the CIS (RE) strategy, which focuses on the temporal information of the sound. It stimulates a smaller number of channels at a higher stimulation rate per channel. By default 12 channels at 900 pps obtaining a final stimulation rate of 14,400pps. With the new implant models CI24RE, Hybrid L24, CI422 and Profile Series the CIS (RE) strategy allows to reach stimulations up to 28,000 pps (2), you can choose from 900 to 3500pps.

This strategy may be chosen when the user has impaired auditory performance or when there are few active electrodes.

Strategies based on the extraction of formants: they represent the spectral characteristics of speech. This strategy has been the main basis of the Nucleus implant since it was created. The following coding strategies are currently available:

■ SPEAK, the input signal is sent to a bank of 20 filters from 250 to 10,000Hz and selected from among 510 higher amplitude signals. The selected electrodes are activated at a rate varying from 180 to 300Hz (3).

Generally 8 maxima (1) are selected and used for N22 or for complex patients, with narrow electrical ranges, slow auditory processing, asynchronous, with significant adaptation or discomfort to electrical stimulation. In this way we deliver a slower stimulation generating greater comfort and better speech perception.

■ MP3000, is a strategy that employs a deafening algorithm based on an acoustic model of normal hearing. It eliminates the redundant acoustic information and keeps the speech acoustic information (2). Important frequency information is discarded, the low frequency component is masked by an adjacent high frequency component (1). Reduce the total stimulation rate by using a few maximums 4, 5 or 6. On the other hand, reducing stimulation does increase battery life (2). This strategy can be used for cases with narrow electrical ranges, excessive battery consumption, limited speech recognition in noisy environments, with great discomfort to stimulation or with adaptation.

■ ACE (Advanced combination encoders). This strategy combines elements of the CIS and SPEAK strategy. It makes it possible to divide the incoming sound into 22 frequency bands and then to select 6 to 20 of these bands with higher amplitude and to distribute this information sequentially among the assigned electrodes. This strategy allowed to improve and optimize the spectral information transmitted per coding location and the temporal information per coding frequency. It stimulates at a rate of up to

14,400 pps. The new ACE-RE, used by default in CI24RE, Hybrid L24, CI422 and Profile Series implants, provides a higher stimulation rate with a maximum of 31,500 pps (2).

This strategy, ACE-RE, used in the new programming provides good spectral information with high stimulation speed.

Strategy	No. of stimulation sites	Stimulation rates per channel (Hz)	No. of maxima / channels stimulated per frame
SPEAK	20	250	6 to 10
CIS/CIS (RE)	4, 6, 8 or 12	900, 1200, 1800, 2400 or 3500	4, 6, 8 or 12 (up to 8 for 1800, 2400, 3500 Hz
ACE/ACE (RE)	22	250, 500, 720, 900, 1200, 1800, 2400 or 3500	up to 20 (depending upon stimulation rate selected)
MP3000	22	250, 500, 720, 900, 1200, 1800, 2400	4, 5 or 6

Table: Summary of the differences between Coding Strategies (2)

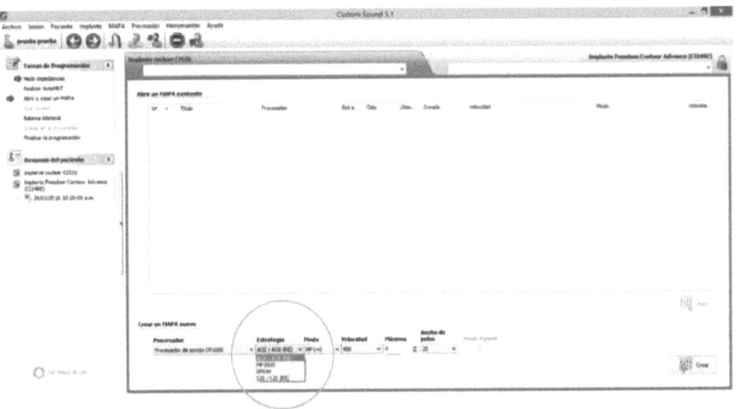

Figure 2: In this figure we see how to select the stimulation strategy for the creation of the MAP or from parameters.

o *Maximums*

The maximum is a parameter of the SPEAK, ACE™ and MP3000™ sound processing strategies, and refers to the formants containing the highest energy level. The value specifies the number of peaks that will be extracted from the incoming sound and consequently the number of electrodes that will be selected to activate and transmit the received signal. (2)

By default, 8 maximums are proposed. They can be modified between 1-16. According to research, 9 or more maxima are required to achieve good performance in noise. In practice, 10-12 maxima are often used (1). After the first 3 months of use, MAPAS with different maxima should be tested and compared to find the stimulation that optimizes hearing performance.

It is important to take into account that increasing the maxima also increases the total stimulation speed. Consequently, the patient will perceive more loudness despite maintaining the same stimulation levels. In some cases it is necessary to lower the maximum stimulation level to maintain comfort.

In those patients in whom discomfort to electrical stimulation or deterioration of the auditory nerve synchrony is observed, it is suggested to maintain 8 maxima. However, a map with different maxima should be tested to evaluate the performance.

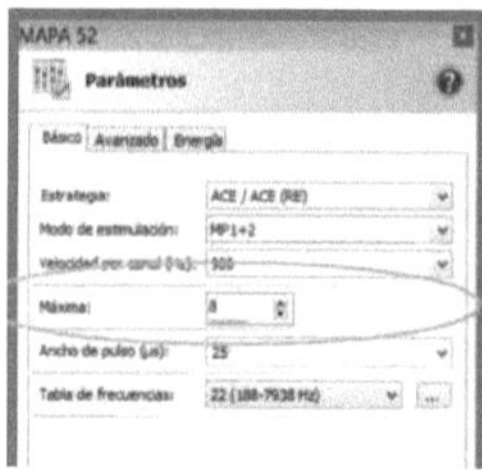

Figure 3: The maximums can be modified from the parameters panel or in the map creation screen.

o *Stimulation Rate (Stimulation Rate)*

The channel rate (or stimulation rate) determines the frequency of the biphasic current pulse delivered to a channel. The velocity per channel applies to all channels of a MAP. The default is 900Hz per channel (2).

Through studies based on scientific evidence, stimulation less than or equal to 3000pps is recommended. However, since there is considerable interpersonal variation, it is proposed to test different stimulation rates starting from the default rate (1).

With the Nucleus24 devices, patients show most benefit at 900Hz, 1200Hz and some less at 250Hz. These suggestions cannot be generalized as this is intimately related to auditory nerve capacity and central auditory processing abilities. It is proposed to test MAPAS at different speeds after 3 months of implant use to determine at which speed the greatest benefit in speech recognition is obtained. We could test 1200hz in those cases with good auditory skills and, on the contrary, 750/500 or 250 Hz in patients with limited processing, slowed or with clear discomfort to electrical stimulation.

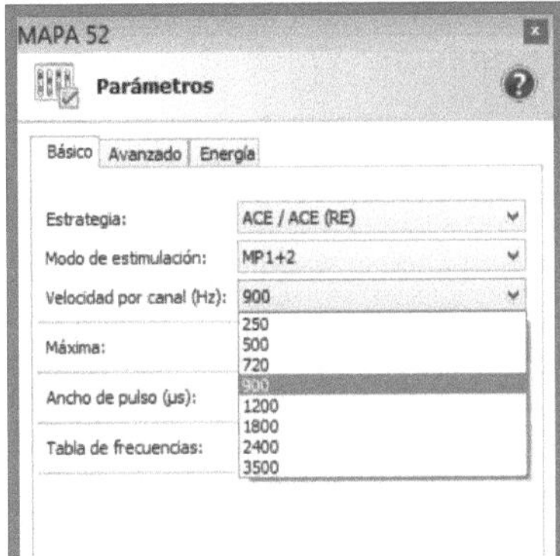

Figure 4: The stimulation rate is selected from the parameters tab or from the MAP creation screen.

Parameters that affect the intensity coded signal

o *Stimulation levels*

The electrical stimulation levels are the most important parameters in the programming of the Cochlear Cochlear Implant[R] . Through proper stimulation of the auditory nerve ganglion cells, it will be possible for speech and environmental sounds to be audible to the implant user.

The goal of programming is to establish or restore the process of auditory perception with good loudness, consistency and comfort, making it possible for soft sounds to be perceived as soft and loud sounds as loud. To achieve this, measured, real and reliable stimulation values are needed. In this way, clear and easy access to speech can be provided for speech to be processed centrally.

○ *Minimum stimulation level / T Level (Threshold Level)*

T level is the minimum level of stimulation at which the soft sounds entering the speech processor are represented. Cochlear[R] considers that it is the value of electrical stimulation delivered by the electrode contact that generates the minimum auditory perception in 100% of the stimulations.

The T level is measured in Cochlear Cochlear Implant users[R] to provide consistent access to soft speech and ambient sounds. When this level is elevated, the patient perceives elevated background noise. To measure it, the descending/ascending technique is used, where it is considered as a safe and reliable response to the one obtained in the ascending technique (1).

In patients with reliable responses and good stimulus detection (older children, youngsters and adults), this minimum level is measured by asking them to indicate whether they perceive the electrical stimulation (by raising their hand or by saying "yes"), in a similar way to the threshold search in tonal audiometry. If they give false positive responses, due to lack of experience or the presence of tinnitus, we can resort to counting the number of stimuli heard or to the loudness scale (soft vs. no perception).

In young children or children with associated components, T levels can be determined with the methods used for audiological evaluation according to maturational age: by Behavioral Observation (BOA), by Visual Reinforcement (VRA) or by Conditioned Play (CPA) (1). In the same way that to obtain a tonal audiometry in these patients it is necessary to have audiological experience in children.

There are patients with great inconsistency in the detection of soft sounds and present variable responses, caused by poor attention, general deterioration, poor auditory ability or hyperactivity. In these cases it is suggested to train them to improve their detection ability and control programming in one month.

On the other hand, we must consider that, in Bipolar mode, the T levels of all active electrodes must be measured, while in Monopolar mode, 5 electrodes can be measured and the value of the remaining electrodes can be interpolated. The more electrodes are measured, the better the hearing quality will be.

On the other hand, if the stimulation speed or the stimulation mode is modified, the levels must be adjusted, which requires session time and patient attention. To make these changes it is suggested to plan a session to avoid fatigue.

Both the flexibility and clarity of the audiologist's instructions and the patient's hearing experience will allow to obtain consistent T-Levels. These minimum stimulation levels should be verified through free field audiometry (1), through speech perception tests with soft input and through background noise perception.

- Maximum level of stimulation / Level C (Comfortable Level)

Level C is the maximum stimulation level at which loud sounds entering the Sound Processor are represented. It is the value of electrical stimulation delivered by the electrode contact that generates the maximum, intense and comfortable auditory perception in 100% of the stimulations.

C-level programming is to find the level that generates a strong but comfortable acoustic sensation. This value is critical for speech recognition, sound quality, speech consistency, voice monitoring, acceptance of stimulation, consistent use and comfort in noisy environments.

To establish level C in adult patients or children older than 5 years who can clearly report acoustic sensation, Loudness Scales are used or they are asked to indicate when stimulation is loud and comfortable.

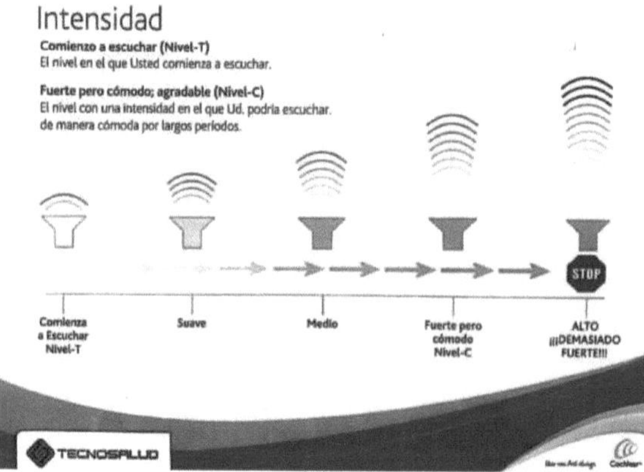

Image 3: Visual Loudness Scale for adults (Courtesy of Tecnosalud - Cochlear)

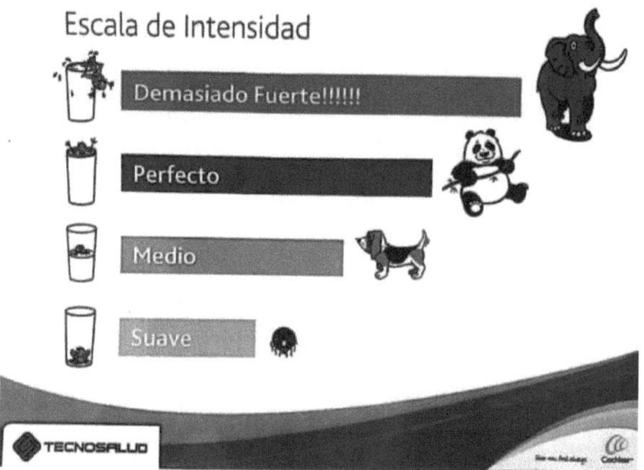

Image 4: Visual loudness scale for children (courtesy of Tecnosalud - Cochlear).

In children or patients with limitations, who cannot signal or express the psychoacutical sensation before the electrical stimulus, on the one hand, the determination of the C level is performed by the subjective method of behavioral observation. Manifestations can be seen through facial expression, bodily change (such as holding the breath, tensing up, playing aggressively, panicking) or seeking containment from the family member.

On the other hand, there is an objective method to adjust the maximum

18

stimulation level. This is through the Electrical Stapedial Reflex Threshold (ESRT). The thresholds obtained are set as level C, interpolate the unmeasured ones and then decrease globally until the comfortable threshold is reached, with good access to ambient sound and loud speech. The C level should not reach the ESRT levels and these can be used as a maximum stimulation limitation. According to a study by Pallares et al 2005 (5), the C level is 19 units below the ESRT and can be used as a guide to determine the C level.

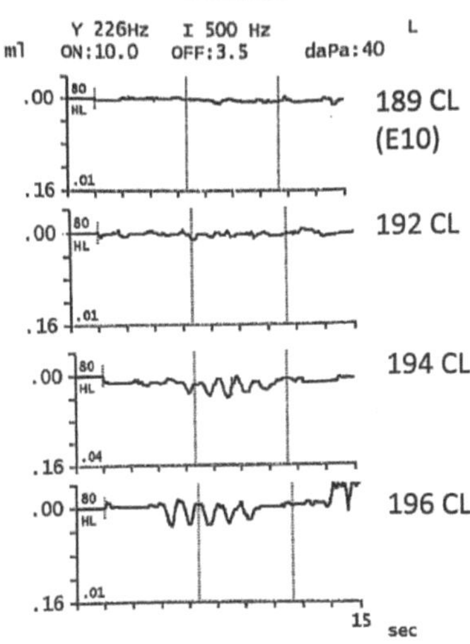

Figure 4: example of the search for the threshold of the electrical stapedial reflex. Hughes M (4)

On the other hand, the Neural Telemetric Response thresholds can be imported into the programming MAP and used as a guide to determine T and C levels. It is estimated that t-NRT, after 6 months of implant use, is at 70% of the electrical dynamic range in most patients. According to a study by Pallares et al 2005 (6), at 6 months of CI use, C levels are 8 units above t-NRT and T level is 28 units below.

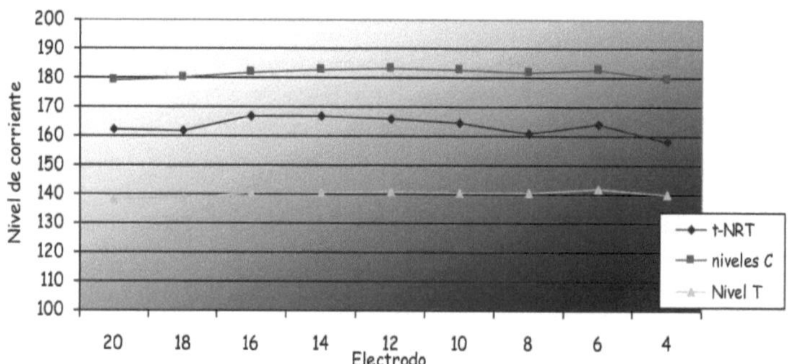

Figure 5: Average T and C levels at 6 months of use of the N24 Contour implant and their relationship with the average t-NRT level (5).

The maximum stimulation will be different in each programming and in each patient, it is a value that cannot be generalized. In the first months the tolerance changes gradually with use, reaching optimal stimulation levels after 6 months of use.

During the first year, in order to avoid rejection of the device due to overstimulation, it is suggested on the one hand that the activation by voice should be done by globally decreasing the levels below the measured levels and then gradually increasing them until comfort and good access to speech are found, and on the other hand, that in the mornings when activating the processor, the volume and/or program should be lowered for half an hour and then progressively increased until reaching the volume used the previous day.

At each cochlear implant programming session, measurement of T and C levels is essential, as use, auditory experience, maturation of central auditory processing, hormonal changes and medications cause changes in behavioral and objective levels. Although levels tend to stabilize between 3-6 months of use, they undergo changes over the years of use.

The Custom Sound Software[R] has three sequential programming methods designed to simplify programming. Cochlear[R] recommends using one of these methods on initial activation (2). The sequential programming methods are:

■ Behavioral method: T levels are measured in selected channels by psychophysical measurements, and C levels are increased and tested viva voce. This method is suitable for patients who can provide reliable behavioral responses to sound.

■ NRT/Offset objective method: the T-level profile is derived from the t-NRT objective measurement profile and the one-channel psychophysical measurement. C levels are measured by live voice testing. This method is suitable for patients with limited behavioral responses.

■ NRT/Predefined objective method: Objective NRT measurements obtained using Custom Sound Software[R] or Custom Sound EP software[R] can be imported to use as a guide for adjusting T and C levels. This method is suitable for patients who do not offer any reliable behavioral response. (2)

In agreement with different authors and with my teacher MA. Norma Pallares, both in adults and children, to establish the optimal levels of T and C stimulation, we propose the combination of measured behavioral thresholds, thresholds of objective measurements of the first neuron of the auditory pathway (Neural Telemetric Response t- NRT) and the response to live voice. Loudness, quality and response to sound are individual and dependent on a varied combination of factors that make each case unrepeatable.

These factors can be summarized as: previous hearing experience, time of hearing deprivation, age at cochlear implantation, time of onset of hearing loss, state of the cochlea, remaining neural population and emotional predisposition to receive the stimulus.

The T&C measurement is at the heart of the implant programming, so most of the session is devoted to it, with the goal of finding consistent responses that provide full and easy access to the sound.

- Manual modification of levels

The measured stimulation levels can be modified manually once they are tested live and the patient complains about loudness, auditory quality or speech perception errors. The bass can be increased to give more body and sonority or lowered to remove the sensation of rumbling. The treble can be lowered to reduce the sensation of a high-pitched, shrill, shrill voice or increased to improve access to high-pitched sounds.

Stimulation levels are also modified globally at the moment of switching on the processor to seek a comfort level and consistent voice perception. See graph 5

In the first months of use, this resource will allow us to set up progressive MAPs to adapt to the stimulation.

- *Electrical Dynamic Range*

It is determined by the difference between the minimum level of perception (Level T) and the maximum level of electrical stimulation tolerated (Level C).

Clinically, it is expected to reach after 3 months of cochlear implant use, an electrical dynamic range between 40-60 units of current.

It is not possible to achieve this dynamic range in all cases. Some patients present limited acceptance to the electrical stimulus working with narrower ranges or on the contrary present poor loudness growth generating wider ranges. See graph 5

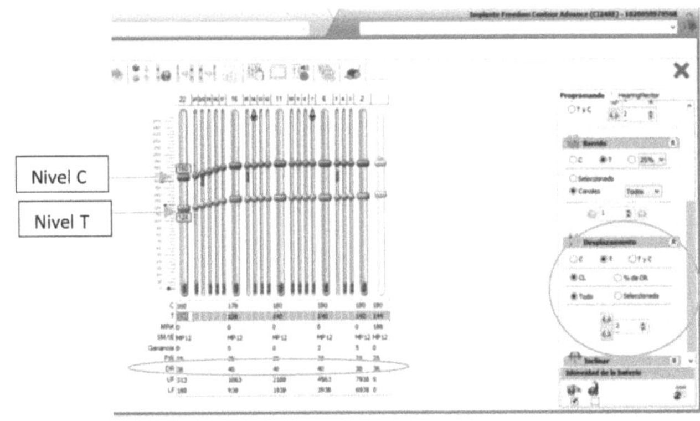

Figure 5: Overall change in C and/or T level and dynamic range.

-Interpolation

The software has the resource of interpolation in Monopolar stimulation modes and between channels having the same pulse width (2).

It consists of estimating values of the neighboring electrodes that are not measured through the values of the electrodes that were measured (1-2). The selected channel is shown in gold in the channel grid of the level adjustment screen and remains highlighted. The more electrodes are selected the more accurate the programming will be to the patient's needs (2). See graph 6.

The objective of interpolating values is to speed up the determination of T and C stimulation levels, given that there are generally no large differences between neighboring electrodes using MP mode. In this way, programming is performed in less time. It is important to remember that the more electrodes that are measured, the better the quality of the stimulation since the more thresholds will be real.

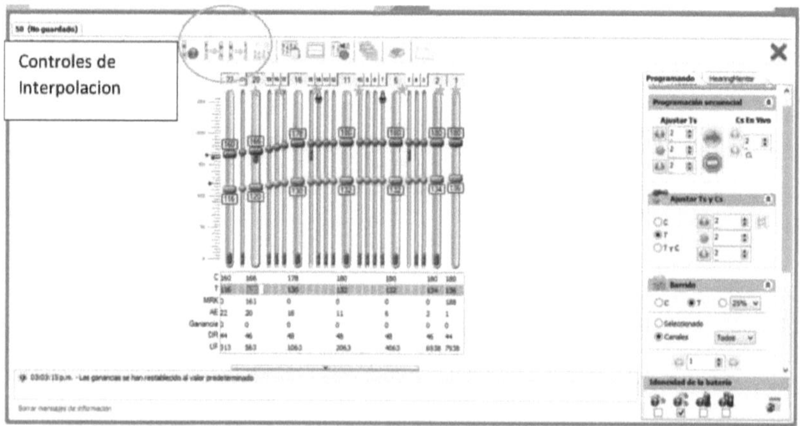

Figure 6: Interpolation of levels according to the electrodes measured.

To optimize the stimulation, it is recommended to perform from the age of 7 years after the measurement of the T level and the C level, two types of electrical stimulation measurements that favor speech recognition and sound quality:

o *Level sweep*

The *Sweep* function allows the sequential stimulation of each active channel in the electrode array to check for channels that are too high or too low. In this way it is possible to check that the levels are within the comfort zone, that they have good sound quality and that the stimulation generates similar loudness between the electrodes (2).

It is suggested to be done in apical to basal direction, at C level to verify the maximum stimulation level, to ensure comfort and at a lower level (e.g. 50% of the electrical dynamic range) to evaluate loudness and audibility (1).

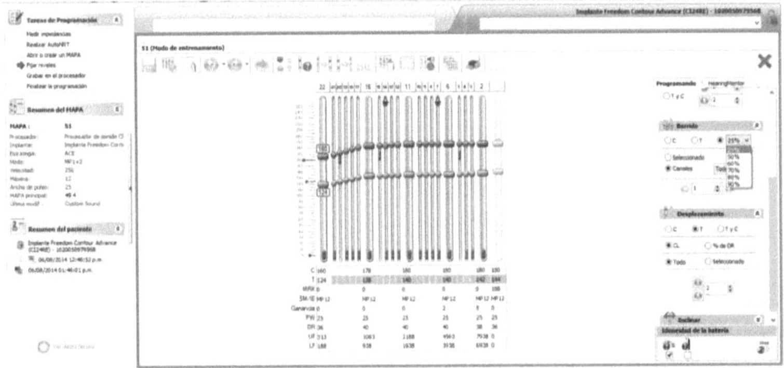

Figure 7: Choice of sweep level, C level, T level or a percentage of the dynamic range.

o *Loudness balance*

Balancing is performed by presenting two or three successive stimuli in an attempt to equalize sonority.

Levels can also be balanced by sweeping channels in small groups (2 to 4 channels). By confirming an identical perception of sound intensity along the electrode line at some level of the dynamic range (2), optimal results in sound quality and speech recognition are achieved (1).

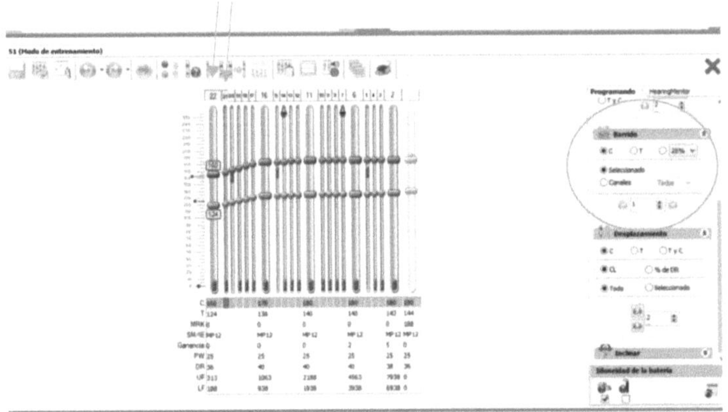

Figure 8: Balance of electrode 22 and 21 at level C

○ **Channel gain**

The gain of the electrodes affects the intensity of the signal before it is processed in the external processor. It allows to emphasize the whole frequency band, by zones or in each channel.

Each channel of a MAP has an adjustable gain control. When the stimulation levels are well adjusted the channel gains are generally not modified, but they can be changed during live speech testing to improve the perceived sound quality of a MAPA when the maximum levels cannot be increased because they are annoying or out of the voltage limit. To improve speech perception we can increase the gain in the treble and to improve the loudness of the voice we can modify the gain in the bass electrodes (1-2).

In the SPEAK, ACE and MP3000 strategies, channel gains are applied prior to selecting the maximum gains and can influence which channels are selected for stimulation. Reducing the gain on a given channel reduces the emphasis of that channel's output, which reduces the likelihood that it will be selected. On the other hand, increasing the gain emphasizes the output (2).

The gain of the channels should not be modified when the behavioral T and C levels are appropriate (1).

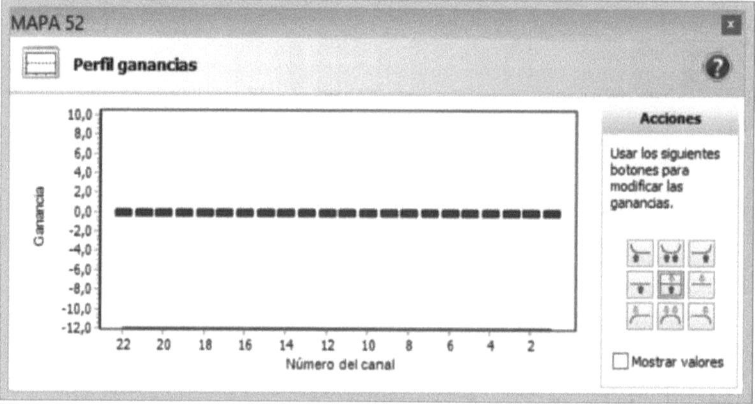

Figure 9: Selection of the gain profile from the upper MAP configuration bar.

o **Input Dynamic Range (IDR)**

The dynamic audio input range of cochlear implant speech processors determines what input signal will be transmitted within the electrical dynamic range of the patient. The lower limit of the IDR determines the softest input level that will be delivered at the Ty level and the upper limit of the IDR determines the loudest input signal level that will be delivered close to the maximum limit (at C) (1). This IDR was initially 30 dB and then increased to 40 dB and in some cases to 80 dB (3).

It is observed that with higher electrical dynamic ranges speech recognition improves (3).

The lower limit from which the input signal information is transmitted was previously limited at 30dB SPL and then at 25dB SPL so that sounds below 25 dB were discarded while sounds above 25 dB are compressed to stay within the electrical dynamic range of the patient (1-3). Currently, the lower limit of the RDI is 20-30 dB SPL while the upper limit is 65 to 84 dB SPL (1). The default is 25 to 65dB SPL (2). See graph 10.

o **Instantaneous Input Dynamic Range-IIDR**

It refers to the range of fluctuations that are transmitted without compression within the electrical dynamic range of the patient. Typically it is 40dB SPL to capture the range of speech amplitude from peak to valley (1). See graph 10.

o **T-SPL and C-SPL:**

They adjust the lower and upper limit of the IIDR. They should rarely be modified. T-SPL can be increased in adults when soft ambient noise is perceived as very annoying, but never in children. The C-SPL if lowered all upper sounds will be compressed and if raised the voice will be perceived as very soft (1).

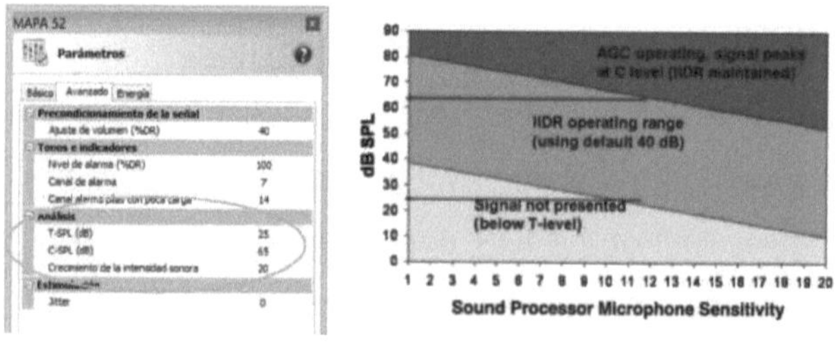

Figure 10: Modification of SPL from the Advanced Parameters screen. IIDR of 40dB. Red zone is compressed to level C. Yellow zone sounds are not transmitted.

○ **Pulse Width**

This value specifies the pulse duration in microseconds. The pulse width can be modified channel by channel using the data grid on the screen or globally from the MAP Parameters tool. The default pulse duration is 25us and can be increased up to 400us (2).

By increasing the pulse width, the stimulus reaches a larger number of nerve fibers and thus increases the loudness, so the level of T and C stimulation should be measured again. In this way, the battery consumption will be lower.

The pulse width is increased when the C level does not generate good loudness and the voltage compliance limits are reached, when the C level generates facial stimulation or when we seek to achieve lower battery consumption. This is more frequent in patients with a history of meningitis, cochlear malformations, auditory nerve hypoplasias and otosclerosis.

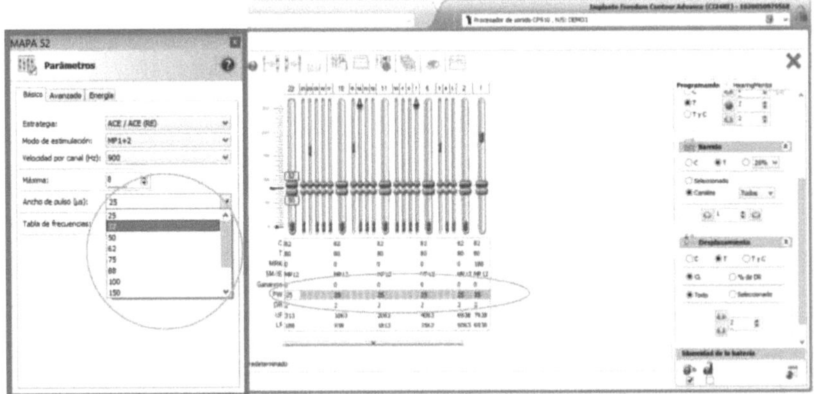

Figure 11: Pulse width management from the parameters tab or from the MAP creation screen.

o *Sensitivity*

The sensitivity control regulates the gain provided by the processor's microphone prior to frequency analysis, thus modifying all sounds in the processor's frequency range. The sensitivity interacts with the IDR/IIDR determining how the auditory input will be placed within the patient's electrical dynamic range (1). Through the sensitivity the patient can mobilize access to soft sounds (3). The default sensitivity is 12 (1). Lowering the sensitivity increases the T-SPL level making soft sounds less audible, but increases the C-SPL allowing loud sounds to enter without compression. Increasing it produces the reverse situation. See graph 12.

It is suggested to keep the sensitivity at 12 and enable the control so that if the patient perceives background noise, the sensitivity can be lowered to 8. If you need to increase the loudness and the C levels cannot be raised, you can change it to 14/16.

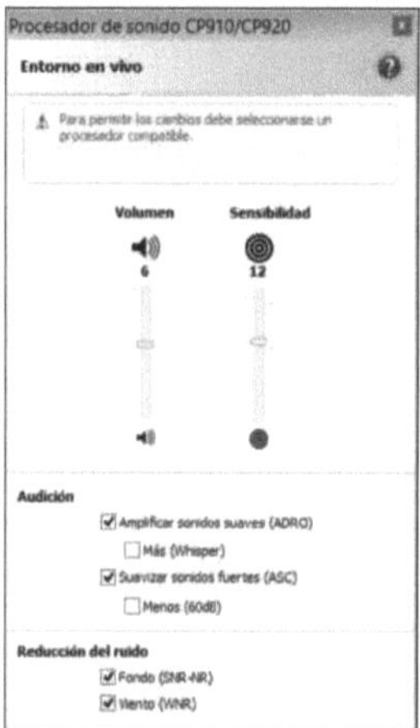

Figure 12: Volume and Sensitivity control is adjusted from the top bar of the MAP configuration or from the program record tab in the processor are adjusted for each program.

o ***Volume control***

This control produces a change in the maximum stimulation level (1). The C levels shown on the programming screen are always the levels for a maximum volume setting (level 10) (2). See graph 12.

The range of modification of the volume control will be determined by the setting of the percentage reduction of the selected C level. By default the volume in position 1 reduces the C level by 20% of the dynamic range (2). See graphic 13.

This is a control that can be modified for patients who want a wider range of volume modification or overridden for those who do not know how to use it.

For a good use of these controls, it is very important to explain to the patient the effect of their modification.

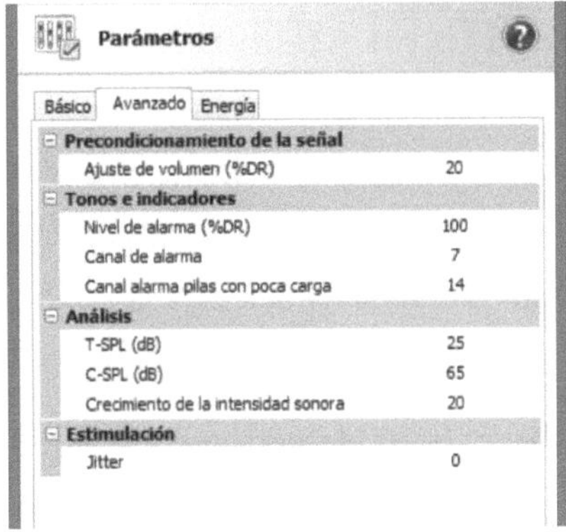

Figure 13: Volume range setting from the Parameters tab.

- ○ **Compression**

Compression is applied to place the wide acoustic range within the narrow electrical dynamic range of the patient (1). Sounds above the C-SPL will be compressed. This provides access to all sounds in the audible range.

- ○ **Growth of sound intensity**

It refers to the emphasis placed on the electrical stimulation (2). It is a logarithmic function that is applied to the input sound to place it within the electrical dynamic range of the patient. This parameter is rarely modified (1). The default value is 20 and the variation range is from 10 to 50.

Parameters affecting the Frequency coded signal

- ○ **Frequency Allocation Table (Allocation Table)**

The first function of the map is to transfer and distribute the spectral information of the incoming signal according to the frequency assignment of each channel. The apical electrodes transmit low frequencies and the basal electrodes high frequencies, reflecting the tonotopic organization of the cochlea. This frequency assignment can be reversed when the electrodes are inserted retrogradely.

○ *Frequency Table*

The frequency table defines the frequency range (or bandwidth) that is assigned to each active channel of the MAP. A given channel receives stimulation when its bandwidth matches the formant selected as a maximum. The frequency table depends on the sound processing strategy and the number of MAP channels (2).

The range of the frequency table is from 188 to 7938 Hz and is maintained independently of the active channels of the map. If any electrode must be switched off, the frequencies are automatically redistributed or, if 20 channels or less are used, tables with progressive reduction of the prepared high frequencies can be used, for example: table 20 188-7938 and table 22 from 188-6063 Hz (1-2).

It can also be modified manually, when the patient complains about the frequency perception of the electrical stimulation. In adults it can be modified up to 6000Hz, but in children it should not be reduced below 7000Hz (1).

When disabling electrodes (for generating non-auditory sensations, poor loudness, failure or being outside the cochlea) the frequencies are automatically reassigned and the frequency band of each channel is widened losing frequency specificity. For better auditory performance the frequency bands should be narrower (1-2).

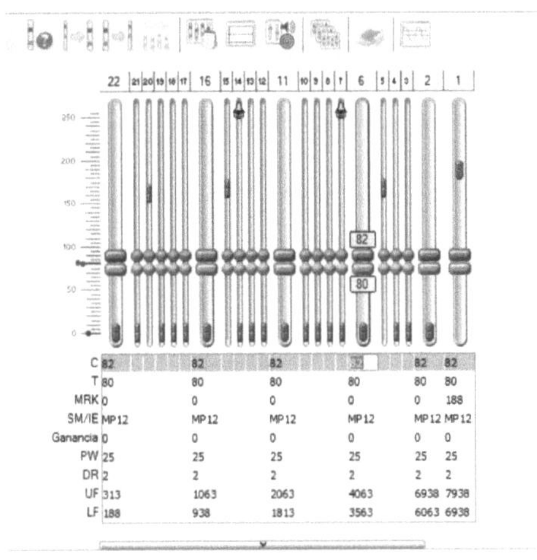

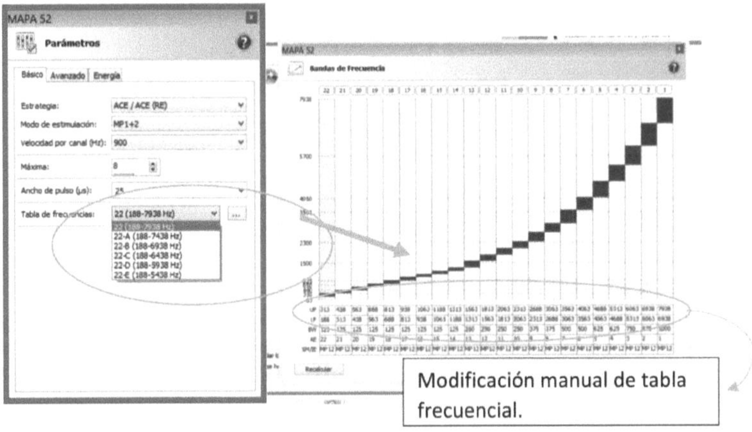

Figure 14: Assignment and frequency table.

o *Reorder channels*

Rearrangement of channels may be necessary when the tonotopic order of one or more channels is atypical. The tonotopic order of the electrodes usually follows an orderly progression of pitch from high to low from base to apex. Channels that are not in the correct tone order will not correctly match the frequency table used in the MAP, which may result in poor performance. When it is evident that the channels do not follow the tone order and there are no electrode problems, the channel order can be changed. Channel rearrangement is of particular importance with the ABI541 and Nucleus 24 ABI implants, as the tone order is more complex in these devices (2).

This task is difficult to perform, since users' hearing experience is generally limited and they have a poor ability to identify and establish frequency differences.

○ ***Duplicate channels***

Duplicating a channel assigns two channels to the same pair of electrodes, and the channels are linked to ensure that they maintain the same T and C levels (2). This resource can be applied when we have few active electrodes.

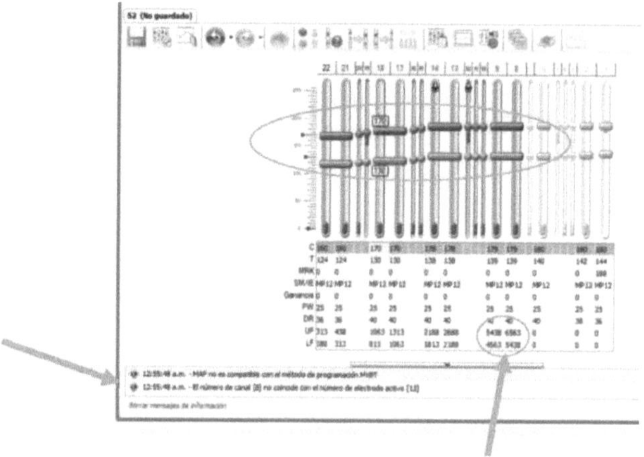

Figure 15: 4 duplicate electrodes can be seen. Right-click on an electrode to display the window with the option to duplicate the electrode.

GENERAL INFORMATION ON PROGRAMMING

o *Protection systems: the implant ID*

The implant ID feature of the CP900 and CP800, Freedom Hybrid and Freedom series sound processors allows the sound processor to be associated with a specific implant or implant type. This reduces the risk of inadvertent stimulation due to confusion of sound processors between patients or ears. The implant ID is not available for other sound processors. A lock icon in the Implant tab of the Programming screen indicates the status of the implant ID. (2)

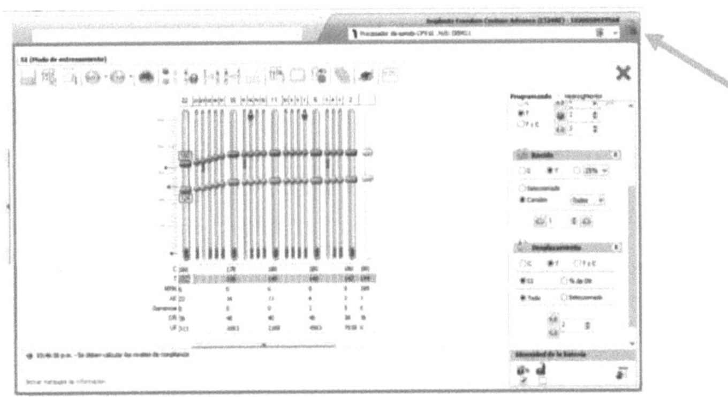

Figure 16: Protection system.

The padlock icons are color-coded to indicate the level of protection (2):

□ Gold: the sound processor that has been programmed for use with a specific implant will not stimulate any other implant. The gold padlock protection level is not available for Nucleus 24, Nucleus 22 or Freedom (CI24RE) implant types prior to serial number 1020050437005.

□ Green: a sound processor programmed for use with a specific type of implant will not stimulate another implant of a different type. This type of protection is for implants that do not access the gold lock.

□ Gray: An audiologist has deactivated the implant ID.

□ No icon: the implant ID is not available. When the implant ID is disabled or not available, a sound processor placed on the wrong implant may cause unintentional stimulation.

If problems occur with the implant ID, the auto-correction option allows you to delete any previously recorded ID values and re-read the ID of that implant (except for Nucleus 24 and Nucleus 22 implant types). If problems persist, the implant ID can be deactivated for all implant types except for Nucleus 22 implants.

o **Mixing of Accessory and Telecoil input**

This is the parameter that controls and balances the intensity of the input signal from the processor and the accessory (FM System, Roger, Mini Mic 2+, TV streamer, Phone Clip or direct audio input) or from the telecoil, and you can decide to listen to both equally or to emphasize one or listen only to the accessory/telecoil input.

Typically, for the school setting the recommended mixing ratio is 1:1, with equal emphasis on each input. It can be used from 3:1 to 6:1 to enhance the input of the adult accessory. See Figure 17

o **Automatic telecoil**

The connection of the magnetic induction field input can be done automatically. In children it is suggested to deactivate this function, since we cannot verify its operation. In adults it is recommended to test for possible interferences. In this case it can be programmed manually.

Also, the input can be emphasized by modifying the mixtures.

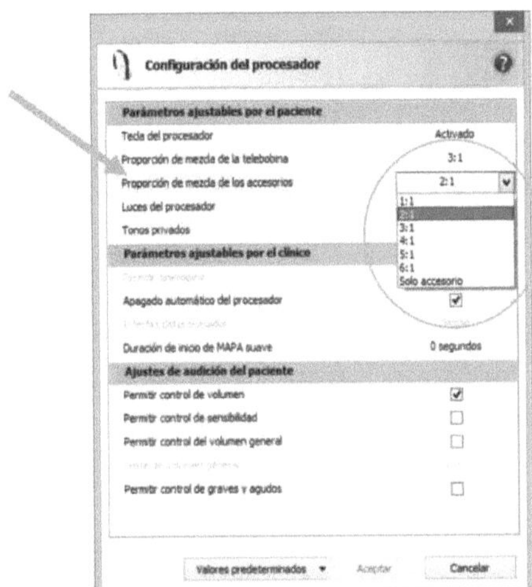

Figure 17: Microphone and accessories ratio options. This processor configuration tab is displayed within the recording page of the processor maps in the final configuration of the program.

o **Indicator lights**

Processor lights and remote control alarms can be activated to inform the attendant or caregiver about different processor states (2).

Permanent orange light: not working

Orange light flashing slowly: some component is not working properly and is not transmitting.

Fast flashing orange light: the child function control is active.

Green light: indicates the program, depending on the number of flashes.

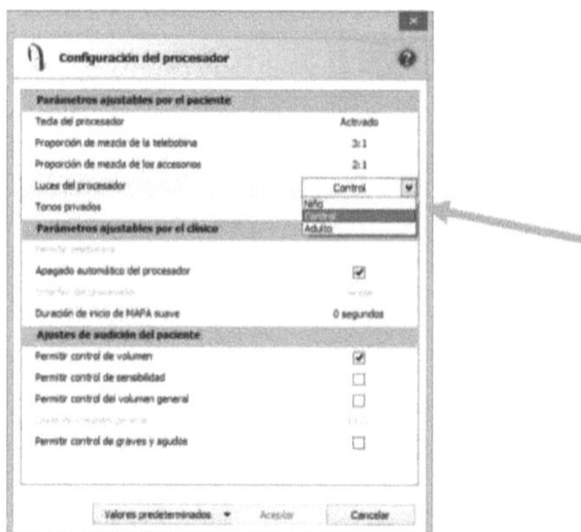

Figure 18: In the processor configuration tab you can also select how the processor lights are activated.

○ *Voice adjustment*

In order to test the subjective and objective parameter settings and measurements that go into the programming of the cochlear implant, they must be activated by voice prior to loading the MAPs into the processor. The desired volume levels are set from 1 to 10 for the CP900 series sound processors. It defaults to level 6 and when typing MAPs, it will also default to 6 (unless changed) (2).

On the other hand, the sensitivity level can be modified according to the patient's needs. It is set to 12 by default but can be lowered to 10 or 8 if the patient refers an intense background noise (2).

Informal speech perception tests are performed at this time to corroborate whether the selected parameter combination is adequate and optimizes the patient's performance. If necessary, manual modifications of levels, volume, sensitivity, hearing controls or noise reduction controls are made at this time.

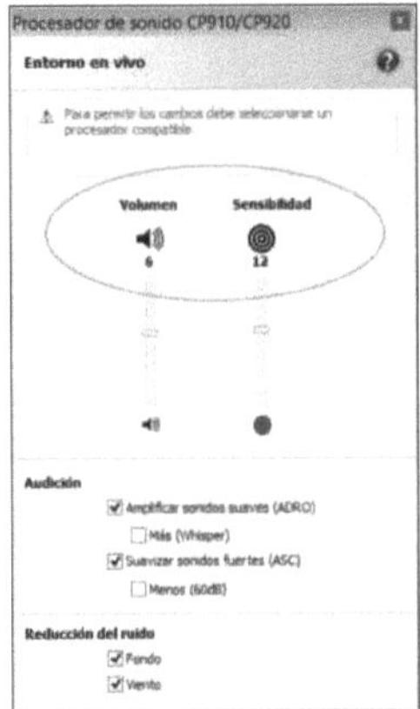

Figure 19: Volume, sensitivity, hearing and noise reduction settings, to be activated later by voice.

o *HearingMentor*

The viva voce test is performed to corroborate comfort, loudness, voice quality and speech access. Once the patient begins to hear, he/she will report different symptoms which can be corrected with manual changes of the different parameters or we can use the HearingMentor automatic change system (2).

It is an excellent resource to apply when the patient is not satisfied with the stimulation.

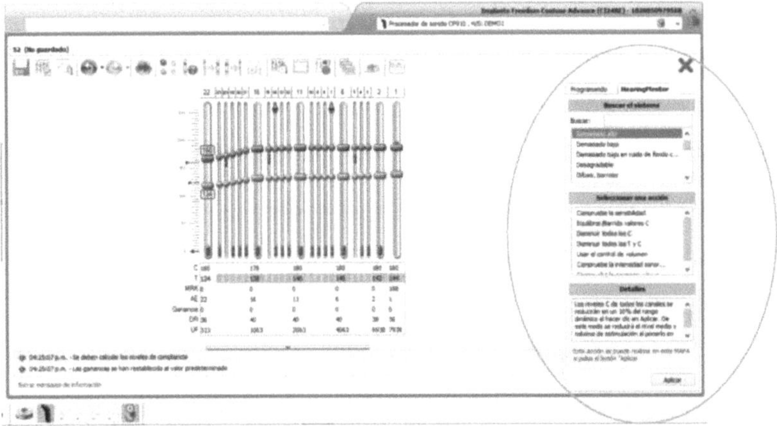

Figure 20: Symptoms can be selected and suggestions can be applied. In addition, they describe and justify the change.

The HearingMentor provides a knowledge base of commonly observed sound quality symptoms, along with recommended actions, which can be applied to automatically modify programming when manual modifications were not sufficient to eliminate the patient's complaint or limitation of speech access.

o ***Electrode impedance***

It is the resistance experienced by the electrode in the transmission of the electric current to the surrounding tissue (1-2). This measurement should be performed at each programming session to record changes in the values and to detect any open circuit or short circuit. See graph 21.

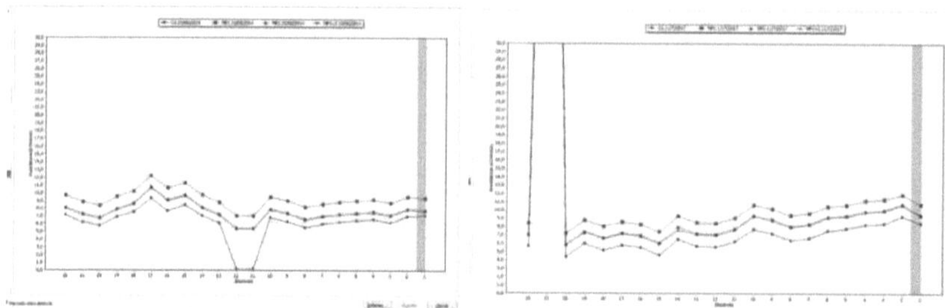

Figure 21: on the left we see an example of electrodes 12 and 11 in short circuit and on the right electrode 21 in open circuit.

S Short circuit: Low resistance to the increase of current between two points of the circuit. Caused by two electrodes or two wires in contact by some compression. It is detected with Common Ground. If seen in MP is in contact between an intarcochlear electrode and an extracochlear electrode (4).

S Open Circuit: Defined as an incomplete current flow or discontinuous circuit. Caused by breakage of the electrode, the wire or by not having a conductive medium around the electrode. The resistance is infinite.

In addition, it is important to evaluate any modification over time since after 3 months of use of the device the values remain stable. Any modification may infer some compromise in the functioning or modification in the intacoclear structures (7).

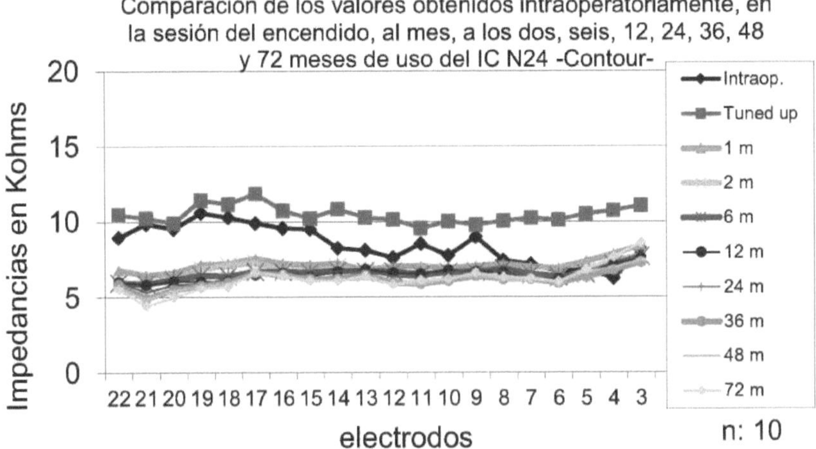

Figure 22: Results of impedance stability over time. Follow-up of 10 patients for 72 months (7).

Impedances can be modified by electrode line displacement, ossifications, fibrous tissue growth and hormonal changes (1).

The electrode that exceeds the normal impedance values 1- 20/30Kohms should be turned off since an electrode with an abnormal impedance value can compromise the sound quality, produce non-auditory sensations, deterioration in speech recognition, inadequate loudness growth and even discomfort (1).

The electrodes, for which satisfactory impedance measurements have been obtained, in all stimulation modes are displayed in green. If there are electrodes for which short or open circuits have been detected, they are shown in red and are automatically marked only in postoperative mode. Marked electrodes will be displayed in brown in subsequent programming sessions (2). See graphic 23.

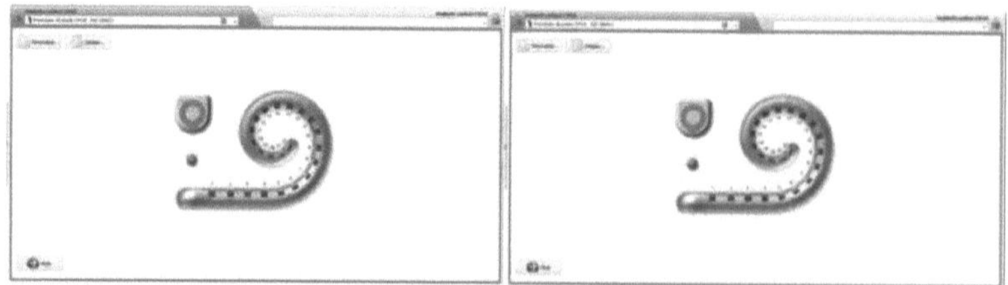

Figure 23: Result of the impedance status of the electrodes after measurement. Green OK, brown not measured, red outside normal values.

Impedances within normal values do not imply that the electrodes are in contact with the cochlea. The insertion of the electrodes must be confirmed through an X-ray (1). See graphic 24.

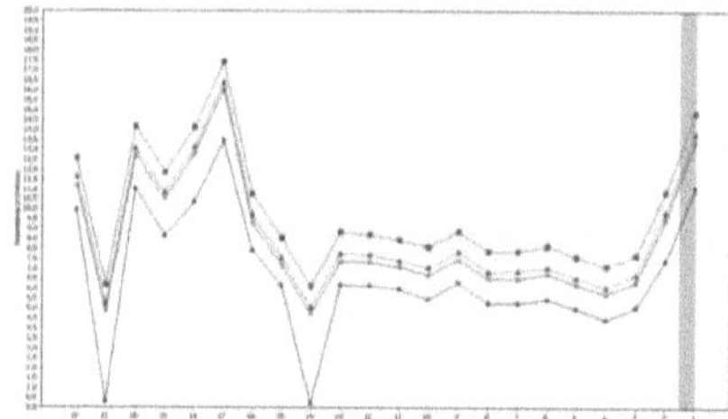

Figure 24: Impedance results measured in a patient with all electrodes outside the cochlea verified by computed tomography.

Custom Sound Software^R measures impedances with the following stimulation modes:

☐ Common Ground (CG): one electrode is designated as active and the rest of the electrodes together form the indifferent "electrode".

☐ Monopolar (MP1, MP2 and MP1+2): one or both extracochlear indifferent electrodes are used in combination with intracochlear active electrodes.

The impedance measurement function is not available for Nucleus 22 implants.

By monitoring patients, we can see over time different impedance behaviors:

• Progressive increase of impedance levels in all modes due to ossification

effect in cases of meningitis

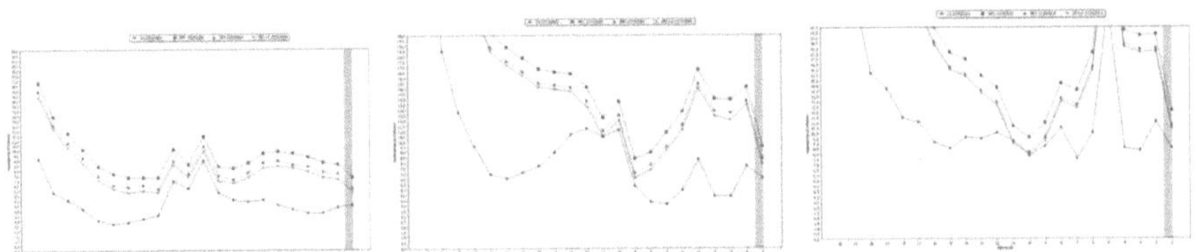

Figure 25: Impedance measurements in a) values in 2004; b) values in 2007; c) values in 2010.

•	Increase in time due to lack of use due to rejection or prolonged repairs.

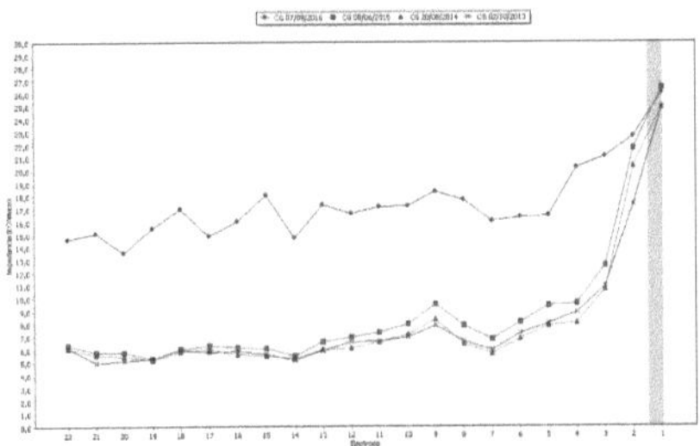

Figure 26: a mode is selected, in this case in CG, and compared over time 2013-20142015 and 2016.

•	Increase only of MP1 due to ossification around the extracochlear bolita electrode or due to shocks in the area. It is suggested to monitor the MPI status and performance to evaluate the need to turn it off.

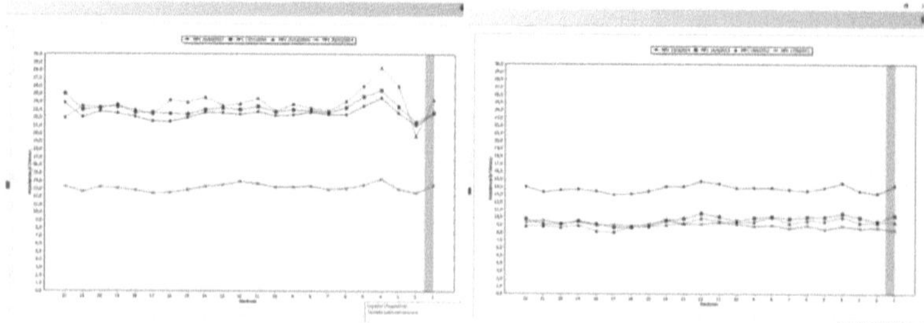

Graph 27: the PM1 value is evaluated over time (measurements one year apart).

• MP2 disturbance: this is a less frequent situation, in which the extracochlear electrode in the receiver/stimulator is involved. In addition to eliminating it from the programming MAP, it must be monitored over time with successive measurements and speech performance tests.

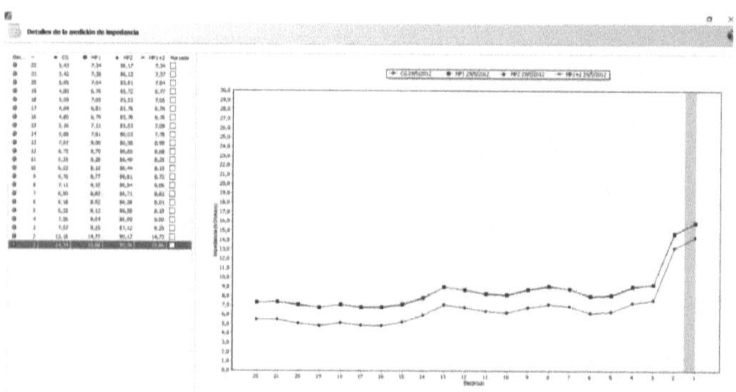

Figure 28: MP2 measurement outside the values after 4 years of use.

• Variable short circuit: the electrode with normal impedance values can be activated, but it must be periodically evaluated because in these cases they are again outside the manufacturing standards and must be turned off.

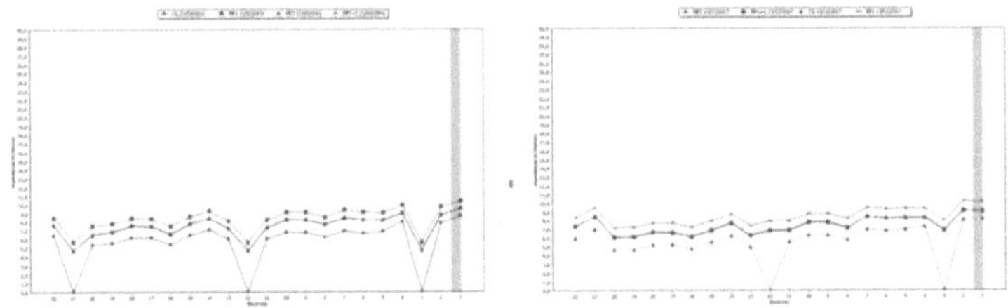

Figure 29: Fluctuation of the impedance level of electrode 21

- Variation of impedance values over time, requires short-term monitoring.

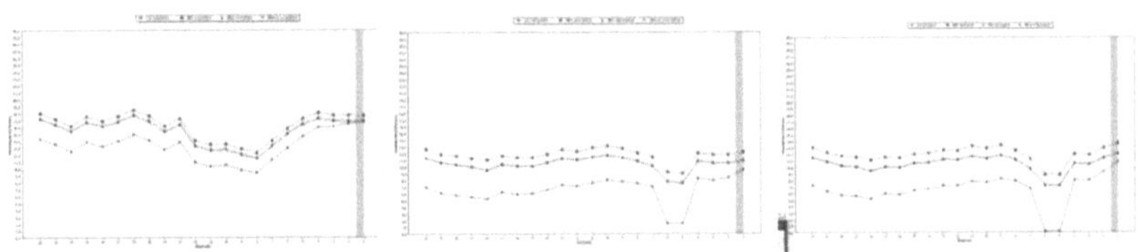

Graph 30: progressive variation of electrodes 5 and 6. 2/2014 Normal values; 11/2014 decrease of values within accepted limits; 7/2015 Short circuit of electrodes 5 and 6.

- Partial short circuit: Described as "isolated damage or atypical impedances", it presents a low resistance of the lowest current flow in the affected electrodes. Caused by small fractures of the silicon around the electrode or cable. As the even electrodes are wrapped separately from the odd ones, depending on where the fracture is located, one or the other will be altered, generating the Zigzag or Alternating profile. (4) See graph 31.

This type of impedance can result in (4):

- No impact

- With deterioration in performance

- Facial stimulation

- Headache / earache

- Noise, static

- Reduction of loudness growth

- Rejection of the use

Therefore, these patients should be monitored every 3 to 6 months.

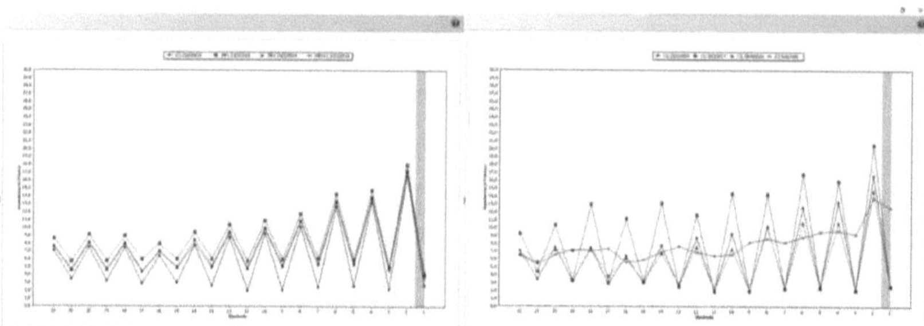

Figure 31: All affected modes are shown on the left. On the right are shown measurements in CG: 6/2015; 4/2016; 3/2017; 2/2018. This comparison shows that partial short circuit occurred between 6/2015 and 4/2016 and was maintained until 2/2018.

Most of these impedance disturbances are managed clinically and can keep the equipment functioning properly.

The following should be considered (4):

- High velocities can generate increased impedances over time.

- Middle ear compromises increase impedances transiently (Clark et al 1995- Neuburger et al 2009).

- If the electrodes operate outside the limits of voltage compliance they cause impedances to rise.

- Progressive decrease of impedance values may suggest a partial Short Circuit.

- Increase in MAP levels

- Deterioration of performance

- pain

- Rejections

- Noises

In view of the above, remember to compare impedances over time and check them at least once a year.

o **_Voltage compliance_**

Once the impedance measurements have been made, the Custom Sound Software[R] measures the voltage level for each channel of a MAP, determining the maximum current level it can deliver based on a power source (2).

The current level delivery is determined by the tissue surrounding the implant, the flap, the stimulation levels (4), the coil, the internal antenna, the radiofrequency transmission, the battery voltage capacity and the electrode impedance. All this determines the voltage compliance level of each electrode (1).

When the voltage level of a channel is insufficient for a desired current level, the electrode will not be able to generate further stimulation beyond that level. Increasing the current level will not increase the loudness of that channel (1). This electrode is shown in red. See graph 32.

This out-of-compliance operation generates higher battery consumption (4) resulting in poor battery life.

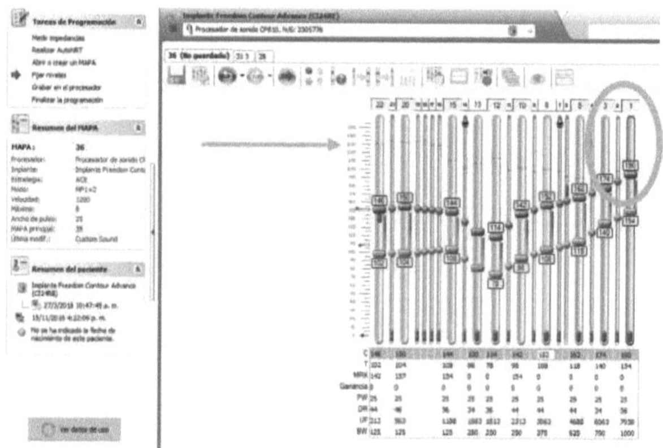

Figure 32: shows in red the level of compliance of each electrode, which is exceeded by electrode 1, marking it all in red.

Compliance levels are automatically calculated when you perform one of the following actions:

- after changing the pulse width,

- the stimulation mode or

- the speed of stimulation,

- when putting a MAP live,

- when looking at battery life,

- when measuring manually or

- when recording a program in the sound processor.

For this purpose, the coil must be in the patient's implant (2).

The power consumption is determined according to the type of sound processor and the type of implant. The Custom Sound Software[R] allows you to:

☐ Estimate the maximum C level for a channel to continue to have a sufficient voltage

☐ Determine the types of piles suitable for each MAP

☐   Optimize the power level of the sound processor to maximize battery life.

If any electrode in the MAPA has a C level of stimulation above the maximum voltage limit, that processor consumes more battery power (4) and may suddenly stop working, with repercussions on speech perception.

To improve this situation, the C level should be lowered or the pulse width increased (1).

If a patient does not use the processor for some time, the impedances and consequently the compliance should be measured. Generally the impedance levels increase and affect the voltage.

o ***Power level***

It determines the necessary strength of the radio frequency signal to be transmitted from the external component to the internal component (1).

The power level optimization of the Custom SoundR Software offers the possibility to adjust the power level of a MAP automatically or manually. It is recommended to use Auto Power whenever possible, to allow the power level of the sound processor to be optimized automatically (2).

For the CP900 and Freedom series sound processors with Nucleus 22 implants, the Custom SoundR Software will prompt you to measure the skin flap and optimize the power level. If you choose not to measure the skin flap, the power level is set to the previously saved level (if available) or to the default level (2) and the power consumption may be higher.

Power level is different for each processor and for each power supply. E.g. for CP810 it is 77% with batteries. See graph 33.

If the patient reports that in noisy environments the signal cuts out, the power level can be manually increased by 10% to the calculated level.

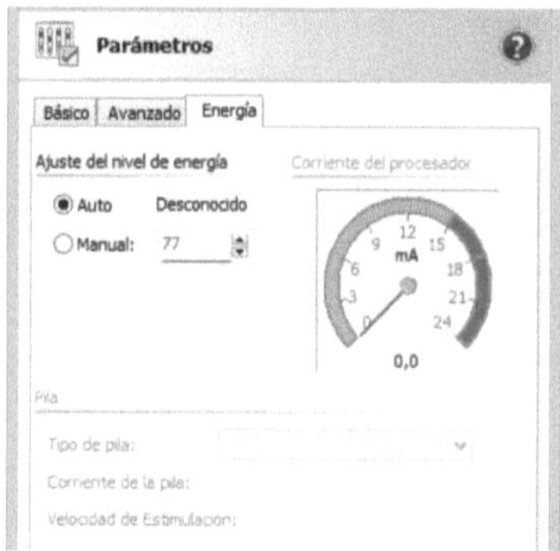

Figure 33: Within the MAP level setting screen, the parameters tab offers the possibility to modify the Power level.

○ **Check battery life**

The *Show battery life* box lists the types of power source that can be used in the connected sound processor and checks which type of power source is suitable for use with the recorded MAP. A question mark next to a battery icon indicates that the battery life should be checked and may be poor.

This information is updated whenever the MAP parameters are modified.

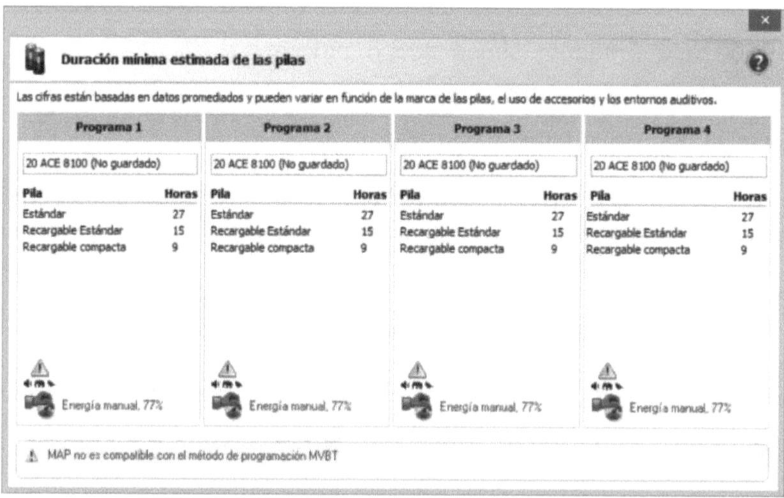

Figure 34: In each case, after programming, consumption is estimated. This is valuable information for family members and users.

If the consumption differs from the estimate, it may be due to battery deterioration, bad batteries, compromised processor performance, impedance changes or voltage compliance. This can be solved by replacing the batteries, repairing the processor or adjusting the programming.

○ *Configuring and recording programs*

Finally, in the *Save to Processor* screen, select the MAP to be placed in each program, then from the *Program Settings* tab:

■ the listening environment *setting* is applied to the selected MAP with or without SCAN,

■ *the microphone directionality* is selected when SCAN is not used.

■ Then, you choose in *audition* between ADRO preprocessing to emphasize soft sounds and make loud sounds comfortable or Whisper to further increase access to the treble, ASC to compress loud sounds or minus 60dB to soften them even more.

■ Further down, in the *noise reduction* box, you can activate the very effective background noise (SNR-NR) and wind noise (WNR) reducers to compress their presence and provide greater comfort to the user. See graph 35.

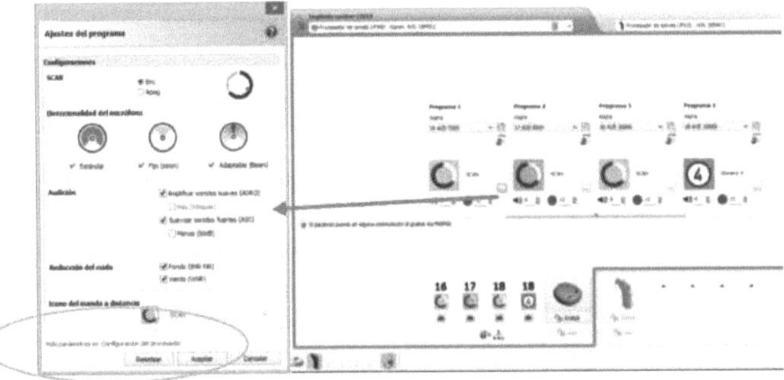

Figure 35: We can see the "Save to Processor" screen and the program settings window.

Then, from the more parameters tab it is possible to choose the configuration of the processor according to the patient's needs. See graph 35-36. In this, it is determined:

■ The function of the processor keys: active or locked for children or adults who cannot operate them.

■ Adjustment of microphone, induction coil and accessory ratios.

■ the processor lights: adult, control (used in adults and some children, which light up when a component is not working or not contacting the internal component) or child (lights up constantly with different flashing frequency according to a set code to indicate that it is working or that there is a problem in the operation). The choice is determined by the management of the processor by the patient and family. In some cases, when the use is partial, it is convenient to activate the child lights so that the adult can verify during the day that it is working.

■ Private tones should only be deactivated when the patient refers to them as annoying. They are used to alert about volume change, program change or low battery.

■ The telecoil can be deactivated when it is not used by the patient. In children, to avoid activation by mistake, it is suggested to turn it off. If it is kept active, the patient is instructed on its use.

■ Automatic processor shutdown: when the processor is not connected to the patient it will shut down after a few minutes. This is useful to preserve the life of the selector buttons and the battery life.

■ Simple interface

■ Gentle MAP start-up duration: allows acclimatization to the sound each time the processor is turned on and connected to the patient, allowing the patient to gradually and comfortably get used to the sound on a daily basis. It is recommended for new users, partial users and people with low tolerance to electrical stimulation. This acclimatization period can be modified from 2 seconds to 10 minutes.

■ Volume and sensitivity control: allows you to enable or disable the use of these controls by the patient. If they are activated, you must know how and when to use them, as well as the effect they will have according to the modification.

■ General volume control and bass/treble control: these are a useful tool for patients with large changes between calibration sessions or for those who live far away and cannot frequently attend programming sessions. One is a control that allows the maximum level/CL to be modified globally by 10 units. The other one acts on the low/apical or high/basal electrodes. It is advisable that both the patient and the family member and/or the rehabilitator know when to use it.

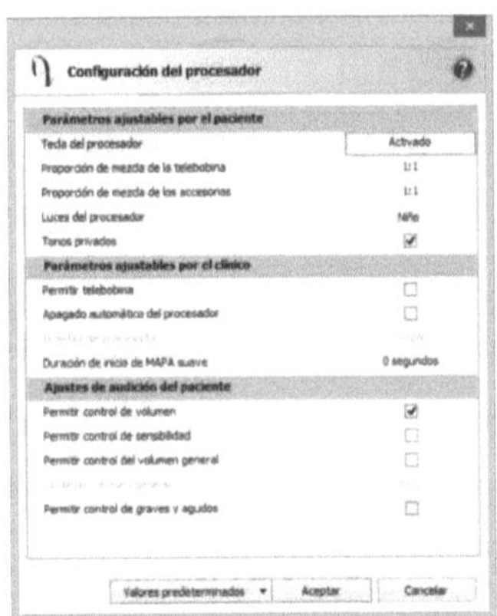

Figure 36: Processor configuration: accessory, telecoil, acclimatization and control parameters are selected.

Finally, the entire configuration for each program is saved in the sound processor. Up to four Program boxes are displayed, each of them with a MAP, an environment pre-processing strategy and a specific processor configuration. See graphic 35.

By default, the CP900 and CP1000 series sound processors, SmartSound®
iQ offer two suggested options for the 4 program settings, the other two
empty ones suggest custom configurations:

☐ SCAN: provides adjustments in response to an automatic classification of
the listening environment.

☐ Option 2: allows fully customized settings for microphone directionality,
loudness control and noise reduction. The custom option also allows
selection of the remote control icons.

It is proposed to take advantage of the processor's capacity and versatility,
loading different MAPs, microphone directionalities, compression, noise
reduction, microphone ratios, creating different programs to provide the
patient with different acoustic scenarios and thus optimizing the overall
performance.

o **Bilateral Programming**

In cases of bilateral IC, the adjustment of the processors must be done
individually and then balanced bilaterally. This last step is suggested to be
done through two interfaces (POD) connecting each one to a processor. With
the global adjustment of the two processors simultaneously and loudly, the
total loudness is adjusted, which can be affected by the addition of the
bilateral stimulus. At this point, the aim is to balance in frequency and
intensity both processors to optimize the overall performance of the user.

If there are not two interfaces, one processor can be calibrated by loading the
programs according to the patient's needs. After having the second implant
with the measurements and adjustments made, without disconnecting it from
the POD and keeping it on, the first calibrated processor is activated and the
necessary modifications are made to equalize the sonority of both
processors. This is done in each of the assembled programs.

This task is complex for those patients with associated hândicaps or poor hearing experience. In these cases, the user must be trained to improve his ability to perform this activity in each session.

PERFORMANCE VERIFICATION

Before starting and at the end of cochlear implant programming, the performance of the MAPA should be examined. For this purpose, subjective speech perception tests are formally implemented:

In Adults: Ling test, vowel confusion matrix, consonants, bisyllables, sentences of the Latin American protocol for precochlear implant evaluation (8) and auditory skills assessment questionnaires.

•	Hearing impairment and handicap questionnaire adapted to Spanish (11).

Amsterdamhttps://es.scribd.com/document/309701610/Fue	nte-A-McPherson-B-Kramer-S-Hormazabal-X-2012- Adaptation-of-the-Amsterdam-Inventory-for-Auditory- Disability-and-Handicap-Into-Spa

•	SSQ-Speech, Spatial and Qualities for hearing scale (1213)

■ in children: Ling test, vowel confusion matrix, consonants, PIP-V, PIP-C, bisyllables, sentences and functional gain through free-field audiometry of the Latin American Protocol for Pre-cochlear Implant Evaluation (8) and questionnaires for assessment of evolution in language skills:

•	LittlEARSMedel 2004 (14)

https://www.medel.com/about-hearing/hearing-test/little-	ears-auditory-questionnaire

https://www.dslio.com/wp-

content/uploads/2014/03/G LittlEARS scoresheet bw.pdf

•	PEACHChing, T.: Hill, M. (15)

https://www.outcomes.nal.gov.au/peach

https://www.audiology.org/sites/default/files/journal/JAAA 1 8 03 03 03.pdf

•	SSQ- Speech, Spatial and Qualities for hearing scale (16)

The assessment provides a wealth of detailed information on access to acoustic speech cues. In this way, performance can be tracked and progress can be observed or difficulties in auditory speech processing skills can be detected and acted upon.

It is suggested to perform:

■ Formal evaluation in sonoamplified cabin at 1, 3, 6, 12 months of implant use and then annually.

■ Informal evaluation by voice in the office at each programming.

■ In children, a neurolinguistic evaluation every 12 months to monitor the development of language skills.

■ Cognitive evaluation every 12 months.

■ Consultation and/or follow-up with a psychologist specialized in hearing impairment when emotional compromise is detected.

TROUBLESHOOTING: TROUBLESHOOTING (17)

In each programming and control session of the cochlear implant, the external and internal components should be checked and partial failures of the device should be detected early in order to anticipate a total failure that may compromise the functioning of the device.

Sometimes users experience temporary involutions in perceptual abilities (they stop responding, detecting or understanding) or complain about malfunctions, intermittency, noises, very soft, distorted signals or very loud speech. Other times, itching or pain appears in the retroauricular area.

It is our role to evaluate whether these symptoms are due to the need for a MAP readjustment, general programming in use, or internal or external component failures.

Fortunately, in most cases of compromised performance, the problem lies in the external component (1).

In this routine control we verify the operation of the microphone of the processor through the monitoring headset and with a free field of 250-6000hz to corroborate the detection of soft sounds. See image 6 . When the microphone is compromised, the thresholds drop more markedly in high frequencies.

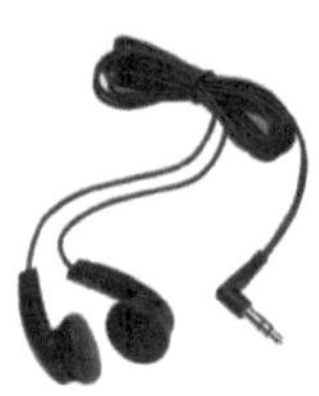
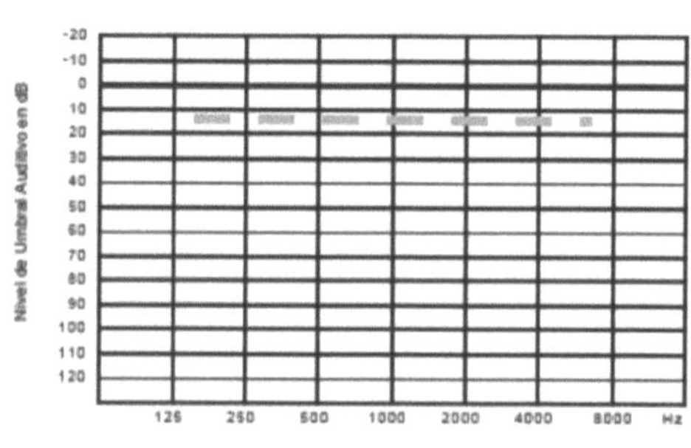

Image 6: microphone monitoring headphones and expected audiogram at 15-20dB.

On the other hand, with the signal-check we control stimulus transmission through the control of the integrity of the coil cable and the coil.

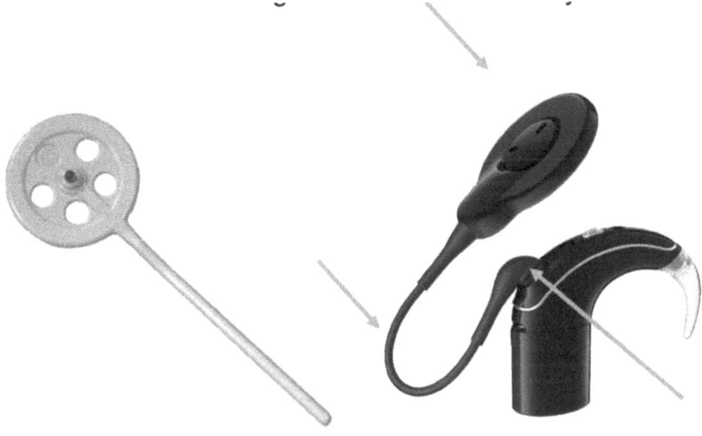

Figure 7: Signal check, to check the operation of the coil cable, the coil and the connection of the coil cable to the processor.

The status of the connection of the processor to the battery, the power button and program change are also checked, and finally, by measuring the impedances and voltage, the status of the electrodes and the feasibility of using the stimulation levels with the chosen energy source are verified.

By performing this component control at each programming, we can foresee future performance compromises and avoid long periods of non-use of the processor due to processor start-up or transmission failures.

The situation in which a patient comes for consultation due to malfunctions is different. It requires a different course of action.

First, the external component must be evaluated:

• Free field to evaluate if the microphone sensitivity allows access to soft sounds in the speech range from 250 to 6000 Hz (1)

• Verify with a back-up processor

- Check the operation of each component, changing one at a time.

When the *cable-coil* fails: it starts generating isolated noises, then intermittence in the transmission and finally no transmission in spite of turning on the processor: It is verified with the signal check. If it does not work, replacement with a new one is suggested.

If the *transmitter coil* malfunctions: it generates noises. If it stops working, it does not transmit sound even with the processor turned on: Check with the Signal check. If it does not work, it is suggested to replace it with a new one.

If the *processor* does not turn on: the problem may be in the internal circuit of the processor, in the contact with the battery or the batteries may be exhausted: In this last case it is suggested to try with a battery holder. If it does not work, repair is suggested.

It turns on, but the *orange light stays on*: the problem is in the internal body of the processor, it must be repaired at the factory.

Finally, if the *microphone* does not work: the coil transmits well, the cable conducts correctly and the processor turns on, but the patient does not perceive any sound. When monitoring with headphones, no sound is perceived or it is very weak. A repair is indicated.

We must pay attention to those frequent consultations due to progressive bad performance, which is not solved by a reprogramming. In some cases this is due to a progressive deterioration of the sound transmission quality of the microphone and can only be detected with the counter-test of a new processor (back-up).

ACCESSORIES

The different accessories used with Cochlear® processors require parameter adjustments to ensure optimal performance.

■ ***Mini microphone, TV-Streamer and Phone-clip:*** after being linked with a CP900 or CP1000 processor, the microphone ratio must be adjusted. The 3:1 situation is indicated for adults and 1:1 for children. In both situations the ratio can be modified to improve access to the wireless device transmission if necessary.

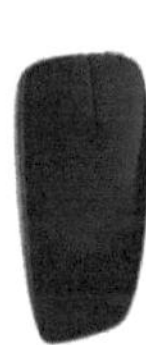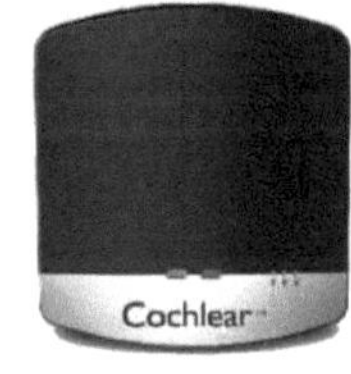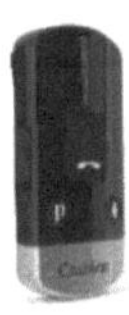

Image 8: devices with wireless connectivity, to facilitate access to remote voice and noise, TV or telephone.

■ ***Roger system:*** the receiver must be placed either integrated in the processor body or in the mini-microphone transmitter. In both cases the ratio of the microphones must be adjusted as with other audio accessories. The connection to the Roger transmitter is activated and the patient has access to a solid and high quality listening experience in noisy and distant situations.

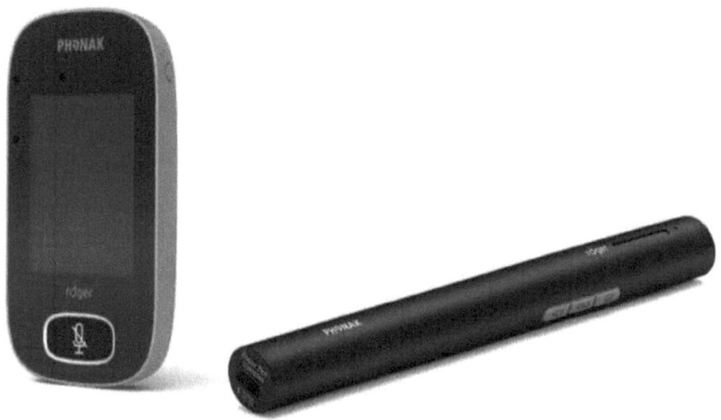

Figure 9: Roger - Phonak transmitters

■ *Aqua+ case:* this accessory, for water or sports activities, should be used with a more powerful MAP to counteract the effect of the case on the microphone.

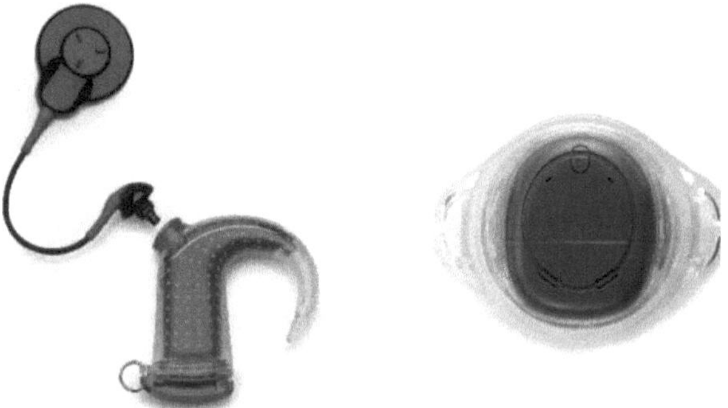

Image 10: Aqua - Cochlear System

There are other accessories that perform the function of retaining the processor in the pinna or clothing through pediatric adaptations and safety lines. In this way we favor the use, support and avoid loss or breakage due to accidental falls.

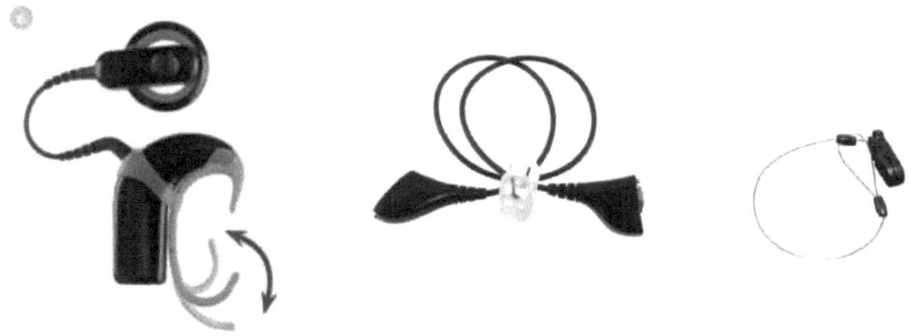

Fig. 11: Snugfit - Pinchfit; Litewear - Long cable for pediatric use and Safety line - Safety line. CochlearR

OBJECTIVE PHYSIOLOGICAL MEASUREMENTS OF THE AUDITORY NERVE

o *Neural Telemetric Response - NRT*

The bioelectrical stimulus, applied to the first neuron of the auditory nerve, generates a compound action potential (ECAP) and is conducted along the auditory pathway to the cortical areas for processing.

Through the components of the cochlear implant, the compound action potential (ECAP) of the auditory nerve can be elicited, captured, plotted and analyzed with the Neural Response Telemetry (NRT) test through an interface and a specific software developed by CochlearR, Custom Sound® EP. To obtain this ECAP trace, through the NRT, the Forward masking paradigm, described by Charlet de Sauvage et al (1983) and Brown et al (1990), is applied to subtract the artifact from the recording (2-9).

This test, designed in the 80's, was improved with the technological development and the increasing experience of professionals around the Cochlear Implant. This ECAP is a solid response, reproducible, reliable and present in most of the patients, which allows to make a clinical use of its thresholds.

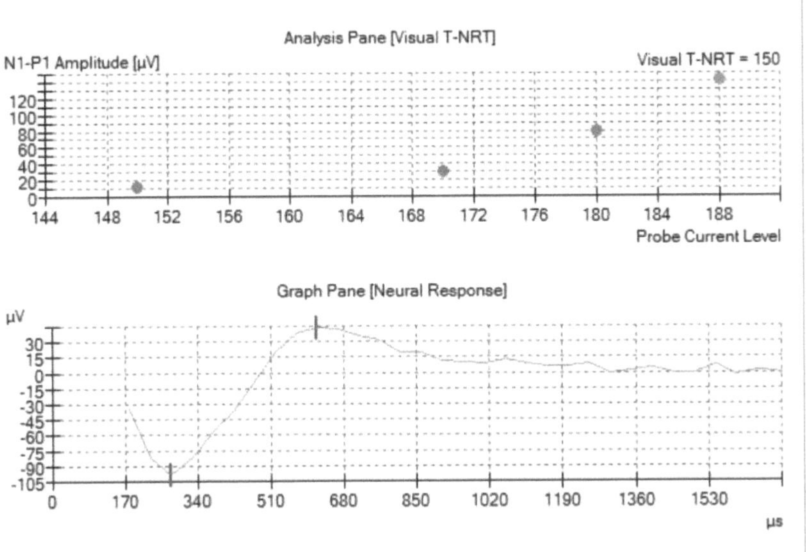

Figure 37: NRT: Top: Analysis of ECAP response amplitude as a function of stimulation level and bottom: representation of electrical activity and recording of N1 and P2.

The ECAP of the distal portion of the auditory nerve, obtained through NRT, is characterized by an electrical activity consisting of a negative peak (N1), with a latency of 0.2 to 0.4 msec, followed by a positive peak (P2), with a latency of 0.5- to 0.7 msec. The response amplitude (measured between N1 and P2) increases with increasing stimulus intensity and is measured in microvolts (ranging from 20 to 2,000 µV). The t-NRT threshold is set as the lowest current level that generates a response with an amplitude greater than 20 µV. These thresholds guide the programming of the T and C levels. See Figure 37.

o **_Advanced Neural Telemetric Response (9)_**

Advanced NRT includes a set of electrophysiological tests of the ECAP of the auditory nerve that are performed by varying stimulation parameters and evaluate different behaviors of the electrical activity generated in the ganglionic fibers in response to modifications of the given stimulus (9). These tests are:

Amplitude Growth Function (AGF)

Evaluates the NRT amplitude growth curve as a function of increasing electrical stimulation. When high levels of stimulation are reached, amplitude growth begins to saturate, but usually before discomfort is reached (1-2).

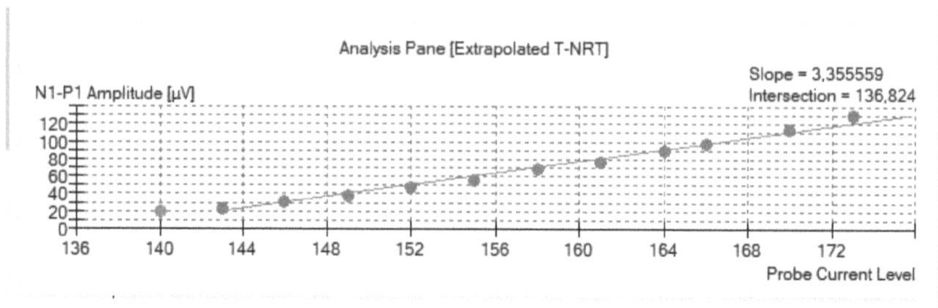

Figure 38: Representation of amplitude according to stimulus level.

Spread of excitation (SOE) evaluates the spread *of* the electrical stimulus along the intracochlear electrode array.

By varying the Masker active electrode along the line of electrodes, the amplitude of the ECAP at the chosen electrode can be evaluated. In this way it is possible to determine whether there is auditory selectivity or intracochlear interaction between the active electrodes (1-2).

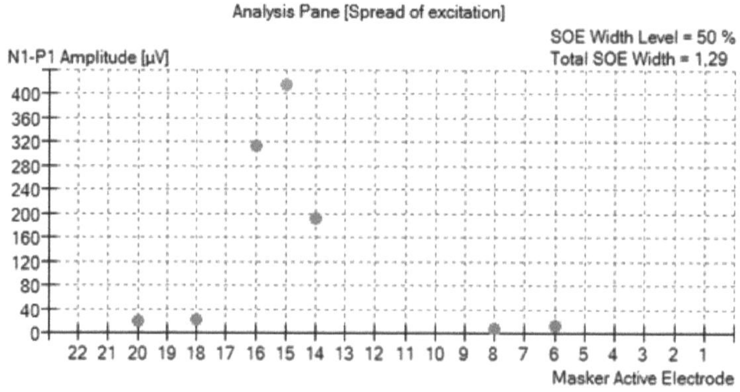

Figure 39: Representation of ECAP according to the position of the masking electrode.

By default, 12 samples are taken for 1'38", where the evaluated variable is the amplitude of response to the change of the Masker Active Electrode. In this work, it is taken varying between electrodes 15, 14, 16, 12, 12, 18, 10, 20, 8, 22, 6, 4, 2.

Recovery Function (RF) which analyzes the speed of recovery of the first neuron of the auditory nerve after depolarization (1).

It evaluates the time of the refractory period of the auditory nerve. It extracts the neural response, relating the response amplitude in relation to the masker interval (Masker Probe interval) which varies between 100 and 10.000us (2).

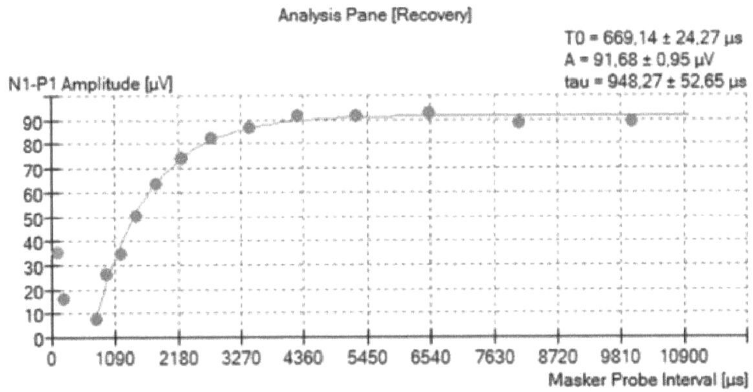

Figure 40: Representation of the different ECAP obtained with different intervals.

By default, 20 samples are taken during 1'38", where the variable to be evaluated is the response amplitude as a function of the interval between each stimulus. The Masker Probe Interval (us) considers the following times: 100, 200, 300, 350, 400, 496, 614, 761, 944, 1170, 1450, 1797, 2227, 2759, 3420, 4239, 5253, 6510, 8069, 10000.

Rate Adaptation (RA) explores the adaptation of the auditory nerve by electrical stimulation.

It evaluates NRT amplitude changes as a function of stimulus presentation time (probe rate) at 10 and 250hz.

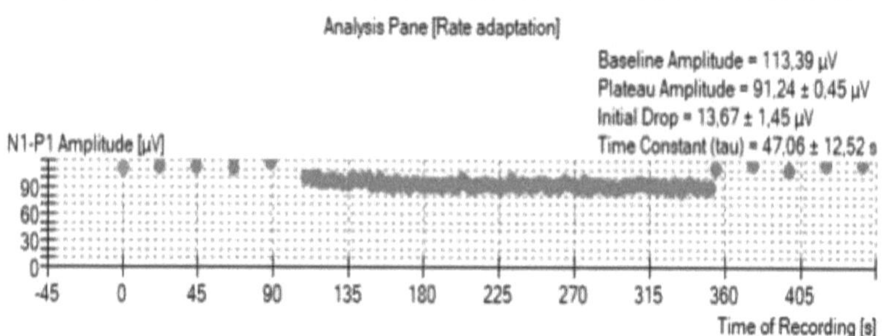

Figure 41: Plot of amplitude as a function of time.

This test can also be used to check for auditory nerve fatigue by comparing amplitude changes over one minute of stimulation and asking the patient for a subjective assessment of loudness (1-2).

By default, the probe rate varies between 10 taps at 10hz and 100 taps at 250Hz for 8'50'.

o **Electrical Stapedial Reflex:** ESRs / EART / eMEMR / eSRT

The electrical stimulus causes excitation of afferent fibers of the auditory nerve that travel to the ipsilateral cochlear nucleus, then to the motor nucleus of the facial nerve on both sides. The reflex arc is completed through the efferent pathway reaching the ipsilateral and contralateral stapedial muscle. (4)

It is a useful tool for:

o Confirm functionality of the device and the auditory pathway at the brainstem level.

o Assist in programming the comfort level of the Sound Processor.

ESRTs are consistently above the C level, so they are difficult to obtain in the clinic. Normal middle ear function is required and can only be measured in 37 to 80% of cases.

There is a strong correlation with the maximum comfort level of the calibration map (4-5).

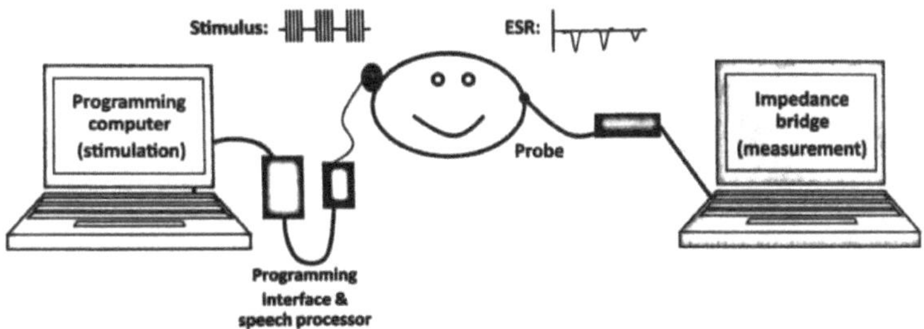

(Hughes,M 2013).

Figure 42: Equipment to obtain ESRTs (4)

o *Electric BERA: EABR (4)*

It can be used to confirm:

■ Functioning of the device, the auditory nerve (cochlear nucleus, superior olivary complex, lateral lemniscus and inferior colliculus),

■ assist in programming the processor,

■ verify behavioral responses

EABR occurs above the behavioral threshold. The correlation between electrical and behavioral thresholds is better with slow speeds. This test alone cannot predict optimal levels of stimulation. It should not be used as a substitute for behavioral responses. It is useful in combination with limited behavioral responses.

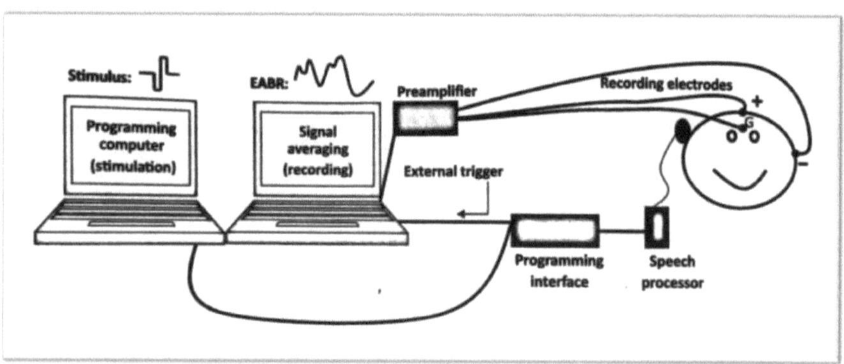

Figure 43: equipment to obtain the EABR (4)

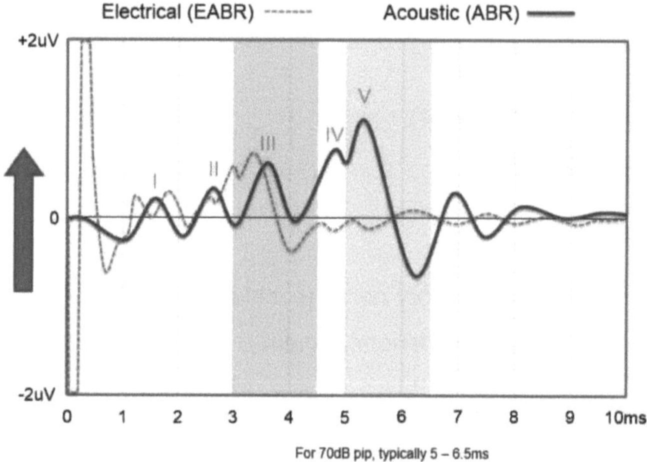

Figure 44: we can see the difference in amplitude and latencies when an electrical or acoustic stimulus is used. Courtesy of B. Navison 2016

- ○ ***Cortical electrically evoked potentials: CAEPs***

These measurements are affected by wakefulness or anesthesia. There are still no studies that correlate results with behavioral thresholds (4). Morphology and latency allow to study and monitor the maturation of the auditory pathway (Sharma 2005) but do not provide information about T and C levels of cochlear implant programming (4). Increased latency and immature morphology are related to longer auditory deprivation times and CI at later ages (Gordon 2005). Preserved morphology correlates with better speech performance (Gordon 2005).

It is a useful study to monitor the development of cortical electrical activity in cochlear implant users.

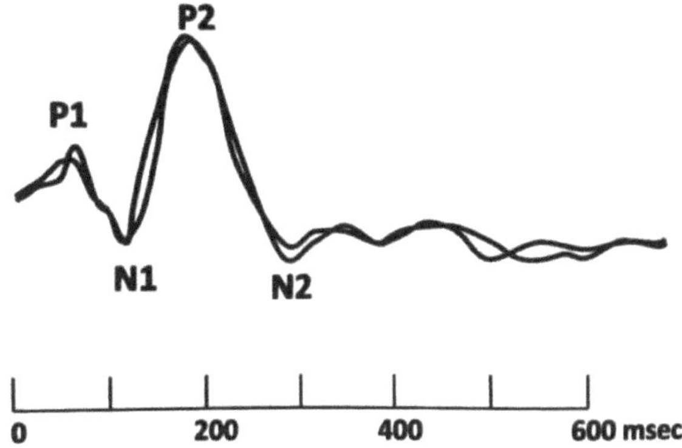

Hughes[1] M 2013

Figure 45: Representation of the electric cortical potential (4)

COCHLEAR IMPLANT SCHEDULING SESSIONS

For the fitting and adjustment of a cochlear implant, a programming software (Custom Sound^R) is required, which is connected via cable or Bluetooth to the Sound Processor through an interface (POD) (see picture 12).

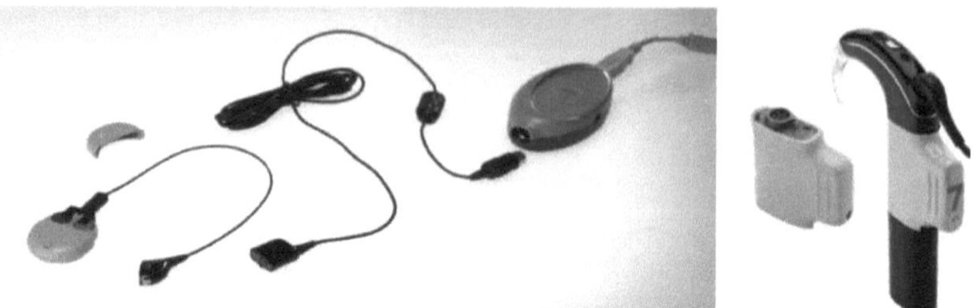

Figure 12: a) POD - Wired programming interface for CP900, b) POD Wireless BluetoothR- Wireless programming interface for CP1000 (Images by Cochlear Americas)

Once the external device has been connected to the internal device and the programming software, the status of the electrodes is first checked by measuring the impedances in order to leave the functional ones active in the programming map. It is necessary to detect short circuit or open circuit, changes in the levels and to evaluate the profile.

Then, the stimulation parameters to configure the MAP are determined and the minimum perception levels and the maximum comfortable levels are measured. Once the stimulation has been tested, adjusted and corroborated, a MAP is saved with a given configuration in each program and the signal preprocessing strategies are chosen, with the choice of scenes, hearing, noise reduction and the processor configuration settings chosen for each case.

The consumption estimate is checked, reports are printed and the processor is disconnected from the patient and the POD.

It is important that the patient is comfortable, in a quiet environment, without distractions and understands the activity to be performed, so it is essential to give clear instructions and not to advance in the programming if he/she is unable to perform it correctly.

The goal of each programming is to achieve the ideal combination of thresholds and parameters to provide the patient with consistently clear, comfortable hearing and full access to speech so that they can use the processor throughout the day for maximum benefit.

It is important to consider that the information presented through the electrical stimulus, although consistent and clear, differs from natural hearing (3). In addition to the way the electrodes are inserted, the lack of tonotopic correlate, there are other important variables such as the remnant of neuronal fibers, the integrity of the central nervous system to process the information, the cognitive capacity, the time of deprivation and the level of acquired language. For this reason, personalized MAPs are made, which are evaluated by voice and standardized tests.

The children require sessions with a playful and enjoyable setting, seeking collaboration in the measurements, acceptance of the equipment and the use of stimulation. Some sessions are difficult to carry out, in others they participate actively and more consistently than some adults in the preparation of the MAP. It is important to make a previous training on the tasks to be performed.

Depending on the maturity age of the child, the response may be behavioral, play or adult technique (2).

If, during the session, we have doubts about the answers obtained, if they are inconsistent or if the child is unwilling to carry out the programming, we should call back another day to corroborate and define the new MAP.

Some adults also have difficulties in defining a programming map, especially those with long-standing hearing loss, tinnitus, poor auditory experience or insecurity, leading to a lack of precision in determining thresholds.

In both cases we must resort to a combination of subjective measurements (T and C), objective measurements (t-NRT and eSRT), reports (from therapists and parents) and formal and informal tests of speech perception.

o **Start-up session or first calibration**

The speech processor is turned on about 15 to 30 days after surgery. This period is defined by the surgeon who establishes the medical discharge for the placement of the external processor.

In this session it is important to receive the medical report of the post-surgical control X-ray that confirms the insertion and location of the electrodes in the cochlea.

A patient is created with all the personal data, the internal implant model is selected, if any electrode is outside the cochlea, it is automatically deactivated from the programming by placing 0 CL in the MAP. Then the processor, the coding strategy, the maxima, the pulse width and the stimulation mode are selected.

Once these parameters have been chosen, and with the processor connected to the POD and the patient, impedance measurements are taken, subjective measurements are taken to determine the minimum level of perception and the maximum level of tolerance and then, if there is tolerance to the stimulus, objective physiological measurements (NRT) are taken.

It is important to clarify that in the measurement of C levels, the presence of facial stimulation and non-auditory somatosensory sensations (SNA) should be evaluated in order to eliminate them by modifying the levels of stimulation that provoke them and allow their use. SNA is frequently found in adult patients with long-standing hearing loss without the use of hearing aids or with limited access to speech.

With all this information, the combination of parameters, settings and thresholds must be tested by voice. Start by lowering the T and C levels to turn it on and ensure comfort. When it is turned on, start increasing the levels until the patient detects speech sounds and accepts the level of stimulation. This point is variable and subject to the characteristics of each patient. Once the armed MAPs are controlled, they are stored in the processor and it is suggested to go out for a walk to confine the comfort in everyday environments (street, bars). This test does not ensure that you will be able to use it on a daily basis.

In addition to configuring the MAPs and setting up the processor, in this session we must ensure that the patient has understood the handling, use and care of the processor, the programs, the batteries, the remote control and the dehumidifier.

The overall objective is to ensure that the patient uses the device comfortably and with the maximum possible access to speech. For this purpose, gentle and progressive MAPs are created, through which the user is accompanied in the gradual adaptation of the electrical stimulation.

In the month of use, before returning to the control calibration, between the patient, the family and the therapists, they promote program changes, mainly maintaining comfort. This point is key to favor the acceptance of the use.

The switch-on is an emotionally charged session of variable duration, due to the diversity of audiological and otological conditions that each patient presents and the situations through which he/she had to go through. The unilateral switch-on session lasts approximately one hour.

After ignition, a monthly control schedule is established. It is common to clarify in the pre-implant counseling/advice that the need for component and level controls will be lifelong.

o **Control and follow-up programming**

These control and follow-up sessions for the cochlear implant user are vital to maintain the success of the surgery and to make good use of this technological device that provides essential auditory information for the development of language and communication,

Controls are scheduled at one and two months and then at 6 months of use. In these successive sessions, stimulation levels are increased until optimal values are reached. When stable maps are reached, level variations are controlled, sonority sweeps are performed and the components are checked every 6 months.

In some cases, after 2 years of use of the cochlear implant with stable performance, it can be checked every 12 months. In children it is suggested every 6 months to detect failures or make early adjustments since they are in a developmental stage. The adult may discover any change in their performance and bring forward the control.

The control and follow-up programming consists of checking the status of the processor, electrodes, voltage compliance, stability of stimulation levels, maintaining full comfort in speech and optimal access to speech sounds in silence and in noise.

In addition, a control of the hours of daily use, environments in which it is used, the use of the programs, the management of the volume and the accessories is performed. All this is achieved through data logging/datalogging performed by the processor and plotted by the Custom SoundR program. It is a very useful tool to monitor the way the ears are used separately. It allows to analyze and interpret the way the patient uses and is exposed to speech, and from there it is possible to make suggestions to improve the performance and development of auditory skills.

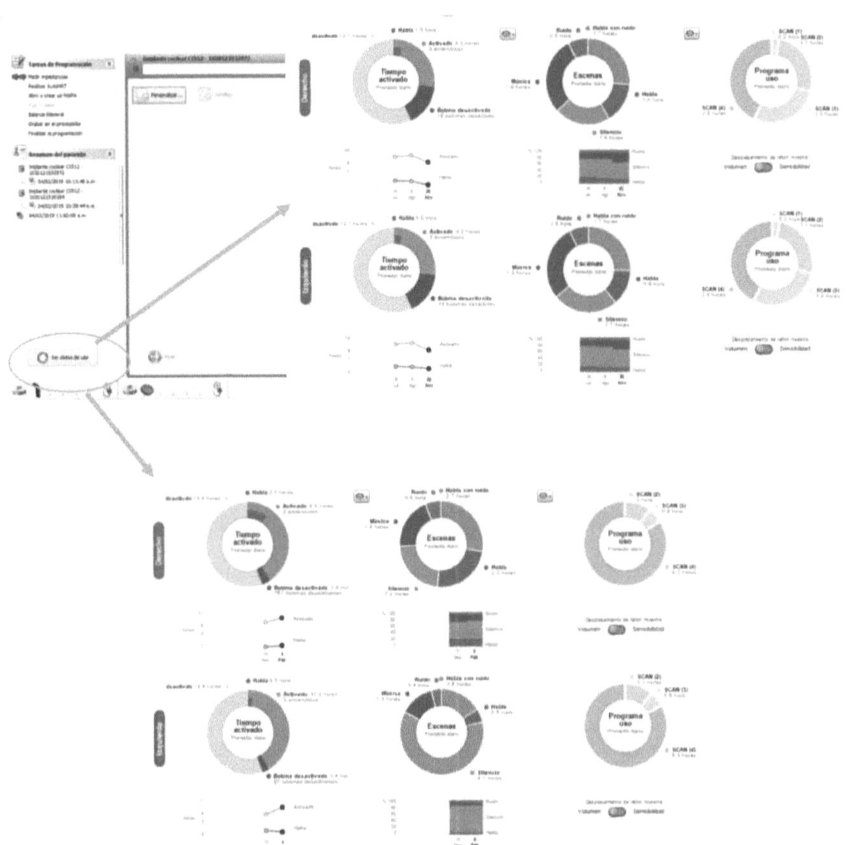

Figure 46: from "View data in use" the information is displayed by ear and aspect to be evaluated: time activated, scenes and program in use. The first case shows that the hours of use are limited with many disconnections of the coils, this is the case of an 18 month old girl and this is to be expected, but it allows us to suggest modifying the magnet or the way of holding it. On the other hand, the first case shows that she was slowly accepting the program changes and in the second case the adaptation was much faster.

Once the program settings have been recorded in the processor, a free-field audiometry is performed and progress in auditory skills is verified through formal speech perception tests to corroborate progress in auditory skills and access to speech sounds.

After the 3rd calibration, different speeds, maxima, parameters and preprocessing strategies can be tested to determine which combination of parameters gives you the most benefit.

The measurement of t-NRT and advanced NRT should be performed once a year to monitor changes in the electrical activity of the peripheral portion of the auditory nerve. See graph 47 and 48.

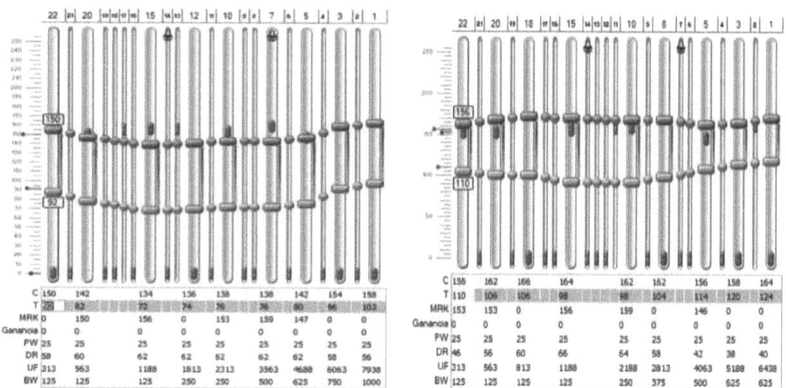

Figure 47: the stability of the t-NRT between 2011-2018 can be seen in blue and the modification of the expected T and C levels over time.

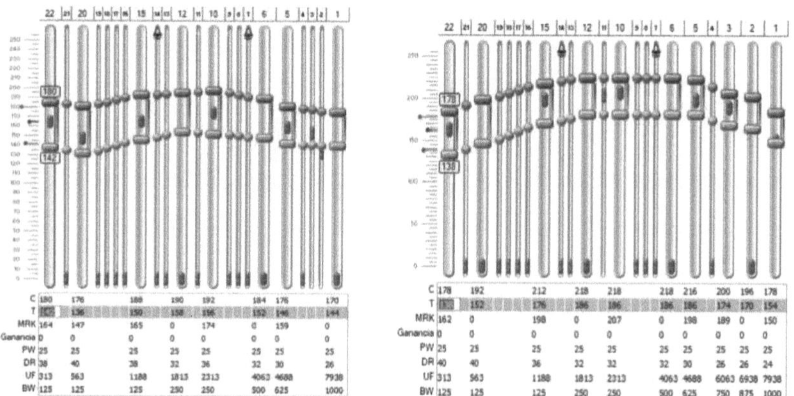

Figure 48: In this case the t-NRTs were stable 2015-2016 and start to increase in 2018. These changes impact the performance which is reversed when the stimulation levels are modified.

In very few cases we see absence of auto t-NRT or loss of recording over time. In these cases we try manually with the Custom Sound^R EP modifying the pulse width, recording electrode separation or we try to optimize the recording. In any case, this modification is to be discussed with the team and with the audiological support of Cochlear^R .

Once again it should be clarified that the precision of the stimulation levels, the speed of evolution and the benefit achieved through the use of the cochlear implant will be conditioned by the chronological age, the maturational age, the cognitive level, the duration of the hearing loss, the previous auditory experience, the remaining cochlear neuronal state, the central auditory processing, the etiology, the schooling, the motivation and the communication methodology.

o **Optimization of programming**

At each programming session the audiologist must make fine adjustments to maximize the patient's performance. This requires a continuous evaluation of auditory skills to corroborate the benefit of the information provided through the combination of parameters and new levels of electrical stimulation. It is important to perform level sweeping and balancing. In this way it is possible to verify the performance with the previous map and with the new one.

In this step, the following should be considered:

S speech perception, through the tests of the protocol.

S listening skills questionnaires

S report from therapists and family members

S datalogging

S the patient's comfort with the stimulation provided

S tailor-made programs according to the patient's environment and activities.

S access to speech in different environments

S language development

S school learning

S social insertion

S use of accessories

S condition of internal and external components

S Contemplate external component upgrades

Each optimization consists of combining the measurements from each programming session with suggestions from scientific evidence.

o **Scheduling outside the control calendar**

The user and his family should know when it is appropriate to anticipate the moment of control and reprogramming of the implant. It is suggested to consult when it appears:

- perception of disturbing noises when the processor is turned off

- changes in sonority,

- Impairment in speech performance,

- distorted speech

- changes in speech production

- pain in the recipient site

- abrupt changes in comfort

- perception of aesthetics

In these situations Cochlear[R] recommends (10)

1.	check the processor and follow the troubleshooting steps. Starting with the batteries, the microphone protectors and then the cable and coil.

2. If symptoms persist, replace the processor.

3. Review MAP parameters

4. Check the use of the Auto Power Level

5. Consult the HearingMentor

6. Check problem description

7. Sweeping and balancing of T and C levels

a. If the Sweep detects any unexpected or inadequate sound i. Adjust the C level according to the sonority of the neighboring electrodes.

ii. Deactivating electrodes with different sonority

8. If the patient continues with the same complaint about quality and performance it is due:

a. Measure at the T and C level of each intracochlear electrode by stimulating with CG (common ground mode) and evaluate the perception of loudness. This allows to identify electrode problems.

1. If the sonority and quality of any electrode is poor or different: deactivate that electrode from the MAP in use.

9. Facial Stimulation: usually occurs in the eyelid, eyebrow, chin or labial commissure. Sometimes patients report sensations before facial movement becomes evident.

10. Non-auditory sensation: exacerbated with increasing stimulus. They generate discomfort, physical sensation such as pressure, heat or vibration. Vestibular symptoms or tinnitus.

a. In these cases 9 and 10, it is important to confirm the condition of the electrodes.

b. If programmed in MP mode:

i.   EF and SNA occur below the T level: turn off the electrode that generates them.

ii.   EF and SNA occur between T and C: increase the pulse width of the committed electrodes

iii.   if EF and SNA cannot be identified: create a new MAP with larger pulse width.

iv.   the EF and SNA occurs only by voice: check the electrodes with a sweep

v.   EF and SNA occurs on more than 4 electrodes: create a new MAP in MP1 mode and another in MP2 mode.

vi.   EF and SNA is not resolved by the above changes: creating a MAPA with low pacing rate and increased pulse width.

c.   If programmed in BP or CG mode:

i.   Create a MAP in MP with higher pulse widths

ii.   Increase Bipolar mode to BP+5

11. Partial insertion or migration of electrodes: if suspected, the condition of the electrodes should be confirmed.

a.   A MAP is created with the confirmed electrodes inside the cochlea.

b.   Do NOT use CG mode. If this is the only possibility, reimplantation should be considered.

12. In cases of reimplantation due to failure of an N22, the parameters of the model to be placed should be used.

All MAP changes require a period of acclimatization. If after this trial period the complaint persists, the Cochlear R representative should be contacted for further recommendations and for the Integrity Test of the implanted system.

In some cases of unresolved complaints or abrupt changes in perception, they require psychological containment specialized in hearing impairment, so it is suggested to carry out supportive therapy until the situation is reversed.

GENERAL CONSIDERATIONS

The useful life of the devices, with good sound quality, is estimated to be 4 to 5 years of use. After that time it is advisable to upgrade the external device to benefit from the new technology and full operation of the microphones and system in general. In some situations, especially in children, the performance of the processor decreases after about 3 years of use. If it is under warranty, the replacement is requested to the representative and if it exceeds this date, a repair or an upgrade is considered.

The audiological indication is made on the basis of the test of the new devices and compared with the performance of the one in use. At this point, a free-field audiometry is taken and tests are implemented for recognition of hysyllables and sentences in silence and in noise with SNR+10 and SNR+5 (where the speech signal is IOdB or 5 dB more intense than the background noise respectively). With this information the application for renewal of the external component is assembled and a medical order from the attending otologist is attached if considered pertinent.

Regarding daily care, it is important for patients and families to know that the microphone filters should be changed every 4 to 6 months depending on the environment in which you live and the activity you perform. This will improve the performance, the quality of the incoming sound and the life span of the microphones.

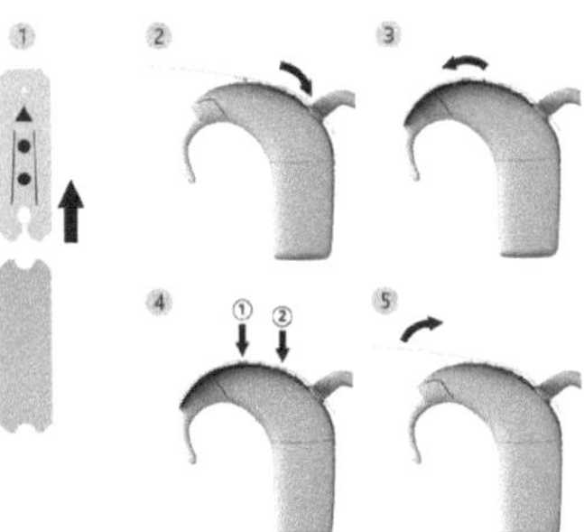

Image 12: Image of the replacement filters and their placement in a CP910 processor.

Of all the external components, the one that breaks most frequently is the coil cable, so it is recommended to have a spare on hand. It is estimated that adults change one cable per year and children sometimes up to 3 per year.

In general, the use of rechargeable batteries or 675 HP Zinc air batteries is indistinct, except in those patients who, due to altered cochlear structure, important flap thickness, stimulation levels or calibration parameters, generate a high energy consumption which cannot be covered by the battery. In these cases the exclusive use of rechargeable batteries is indicated.

In relation to cleaning, it is important to emphasize the need to keep the equipment free of dust and humidity, especially in the connection of the processor with the battery/battery holder and the magnet thread. In the case of the processor out of the ear without cable, these inconveniences diminish.

All processors should be placed in the dehumidifier every night maintaining the 2 month shelf life of the dehumidifier tablets.

As with any electronic device, it is essential to keep it away from extreme temperatures, humidity, water and to avoid knocks or drops.

This care will prolong the life and stimulation quality of the equipment. The user should be instructed on the importance of maintaining each component in good condition. Ultimately, everything will impact hearing performance.

WARNINGS AND CAUTIONS

o **_Medical-surgical procedures_**

Cochlear implant users should talk to their physician before undergoing any major clinical procedure as there are medical treatments that generate induction currents and may cause tissue damage or permanent damage to the internal implant (10).

• Electrosurgery Electrosurgical instruments are capable of generating inductive radiofrequency currents that can flow through the electrode assembly. Monopolar electrosurgical instruments should not be used. Bipolar instruments can be used

• Medical or therapeutic diathermy: electromagnetic radiation cannot be used on the head or neck.

• Neurostimulation: do not use on cochlear implant.

• Electroconvulsive therapy: do not use under any circumstances.

• Ionizing radiation therapy: do not use directly on the implant.

o **_Magnetic Resonance Imaging (MRI)_**

In principle, this study is contraindicated for the patient with a cochlear implant. Neither can he/she stay in a room where there is an MRI machine unless the processor is removed from his/her head.

The image quality will be affected by the cochlear implant up to 11 cm from the implant and this shadowing reduces the diagnostic information around the implant.

If the study is necessary, the patient can undergo it taking into account some safety indications depending on the implant model and the power of the resonance, see the table below (10):

Nucleus ʀ 24 Series

More than 1.5 teslas (T) up to 3 T, inclusive	Surgically remove the magnet
Over 0.2 T up to 1.5 T inclusive	Do not remove the magnet for the magnetic resonance imaging, bandaging the head of the patient to ensure that the magnet will not move.
0.2 T or less	Do not remove the magnet for MRI No bandage necessary

Nucleus ʀ 22 series with removable magnet	
Up to 1.5 T	remove the magnet surgically
Nucleus ʀ 22 series WITHOUT magnet removable	magnetic resonance imaging is contraindicated

○ ***Ingestion of small parts or batteries***

Parents and caregivers should be reminded that these components are dangerous if ingested. Therefore, keep out of reach of children. If swallowed, seek medical attention at the nearest emergency room.

○ ***Head trauma***

A blow to the head in the area of the cochlear implant can damage its internal components and cause its failure. In this situation it is advisable to attend a medical and audiological control to corroborate the state and functioning of the components.

Any sharp injury in the area of the internal receptor can induce an infection. For this reason it is necessary to go immediately for a check-up with the otologist.

○ **Abrupt changes in hearing quality**

If you notice significant changes in sound quality or unpleasant sound, disconnect your processor and contact the implant center for audiological and medical follow-up.

○ **Use of another processor**

Each processor is programmed specifically for each individual. You cannot use another person's processor as you may sometimes perceive the sound to be distorted or too loud. It is contraindicated to use processors that are set for another person. The new implant models are protected so that they will not work if placed in another patient or in the wrong ear.

○ **Extreme temperatures**

Do not use the processor at temperatures above +40 °C or + 104 °F or below + 5 °C or +41 °F and do not store the processor at temperatures above +50 °C or +122 °F, or below -20 °C or -4 °F.

○ **Transmission towers**

The sound quality of the processor may be intermittently distorted when you are approximately 1.6 km or 1 mile from a radio or TV transmission tower. This effect is temporary and will not damage the processor.

Interference may occur in the vicinity of radio frequency equipment with this symbol:

Electromagnetic fields transmitted from radio bases, telephone stations, A.M. and FM amateur radio and TV cannot be accurately predicted. As a hint about these electromagnetic fields, it should be considered that the processor that is above an exceeded level of radio frequency may present an abnormal performance. Above the range of 150 KHz to 80 MHz the magnetic field should be less than 3V/m. If you perceive temporary noise or interference that subsides when you move away from this zone, it is suggested to consult your audiologist and Cochlear representative. [R]

o **Alarm systems and metal detectors**

These devices produce strong electromagnetic fields. Some patients may experience sound distortion when passing through or near these devices. For this reason, patients should avoid them and should wear their user identification card. If they pass through them they may hear a buzzing or distorted sound temporarily.

o **Batteries**

Cochlear[R] does not recommend the use of alkaline or silver oxide batteries as they can increase the temperature and cause severe burns and damage to the processor. It ONLY recommends the use of zinc air batteries as they are safe.

o **Rechargeable batteries**

In certain circumstances they can become hot and cause damage to the skin, so if this temperature increase is detected you should remove them immediately and contact your clinician and your CochlearR representative.

In small children or children with limited motor skills, the temperature of the rechargeable batteries must be controlled by the caregivers.

These should not be worn under clothing. When using fasteners evaluate the possibility of removing the processor by the patient if he/she detects this increase in temperature.

o **Diving**

The immersion depth is determined by the internal implant model:

Type of implant	Maximum depth
Nucleus Freedom and CI500 Series	40 m / 131 ft
Nucleus 24 and Nucleus 22 series	25 m/ 81 ft

o **_Sound_**

It is recommended not to use the processor while the patient is sleeping as it cannot detect if the battery temperature rises.

o **_Remote assistant or remote control_**

Because it emits electromagnetic energy, it may interfere when in close proximity to other medical devices such as pacemakers or implanted defibrillators. It is therefore recommended that the remote assistant be more than 15 cm or 6 inches away.

BIBLIOGRAPHY

1. Wolfe, Jace; Schafer, Erin Programming Cochlear Implants. Plural Publishing 2010

2. Cochlear Software Custom Sound version 4.4 User Guide. Cochlear Limited 2016

3. Manrique, M.; Huarte, A. Cochlear implants Masson 2003.

4. Hughes M Objective Measures in Cochlear Implants- Plural Publishing 2013.

5. Pallares, N.; Diamante, V.; Giraudo, E.; Fanelli, K. Relationship of postoperative ESRT to behavioral levels in children implanted with the Nucleus 24 Cochlear System. 10th Symposium on Cochlear Implants in children. Dallas 2005.

6. Pallares, N.; Diamante, V.; Fanelli, K. Intraoperative t-NRT and subjective levels in children implanted with the N24 Cochlear Implant System. 10th Symposium on Cochlear Implants in children. Dallas 2005.

7. Pallares, N.; Fanelli K.; Diamante, V. Electrode Impedance up to 72 months of CI use in children with Contour electrode - 11th European Symposium on Paediatric Cochlear Implantation - Istanbul - 2013.

8. Latin American Cochlear Pre-Implant Evaluation Protocol - CochlearR www.pkasesorias.cl/PDF/PROTOCOLO LATIN AMERICAN EV.

9. Fanelli, K. Advanced Neural Telemetric Response in postlingual adults with Cochlear Implant- Final Integrative Work - Universidad del Museo Social Argentino - 2016.

10. Clinical Guidance Document. CochlearTM Cochlear Software Custom Sound version 5.1

11. Fuente, A., McPherson, B., Kramer, S., & Hormazàbal, X. Adaptation of the Amsterdam Inventory for Auditory Disability and Handicap Into Spanish -

Disability & Rehabilitation, 2012; 34(24): 2076-2084 © 2012 Informa UK.

12. Juan Zhang, Richard Tyler,b Haihong Ji, Camille Dunn, Ningyu Wang, Marlan Hansen, and Bruce Gantz - Speech, Spatial and Qualities of Hearing Scale (SSQ) and Spatial Hearing Questionnaire (SHQ) Changes Over Time in Adults With Simultaneous Cochlear Implants - American Journal of Audiology - Vol. 24 - 384-397 - September 2015.

13. Gatehouse, Stuart and Noble, William - The Speech, Spatial and Qualities of Hearing Scale (SSQ)- International journal of audiology - March 2004 Vol 43 85-99

14. Medel LittlEARS hearing questionnaire for children 2004

15. Ching, T.; Hill, M. The Parents' Evaluation of Aural/Oral Performance of Children (PEACH) Scale: Normative Data J Am Acad Audiol 18:220-235 (2007).

16. Galvin, Karyn & Noble, William. Adaptation of the speech, spatial, and qualities of hearing scale for use with children, parents, and teachers. Cochlear implants international. 14. 2013

17. Diamante, V.: Pallares, N. Cochlear Implant - in process of editing/printing

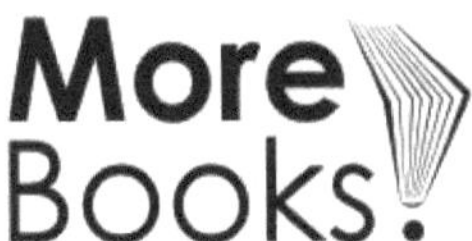

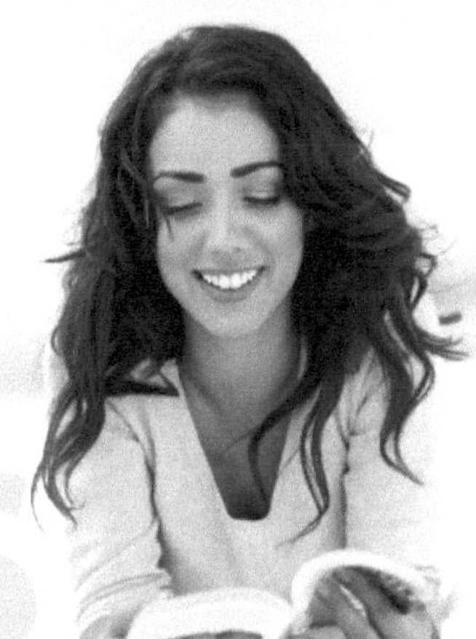

I want morebooks!

Buy your books fast and straightforward online - at one of world's fastest growing online book stores! Environmentally sound due to Print-on-Demand technologies.

Buy your books online at
www.morebooks.shop

Kaufen Sie Ihre Bücher schnell und unkompliziert online – auf einer der am schnellsten wachsenden Buchhandelsplattformen weltweit! Dank Print-On-Demand umwelt- und ressourcenschonend produzi ert.

Bücher schneller online kaufen
www.morebooks.shop

info@omniscriptum.com
www.omniscriptum.com

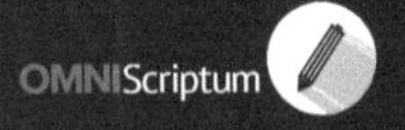

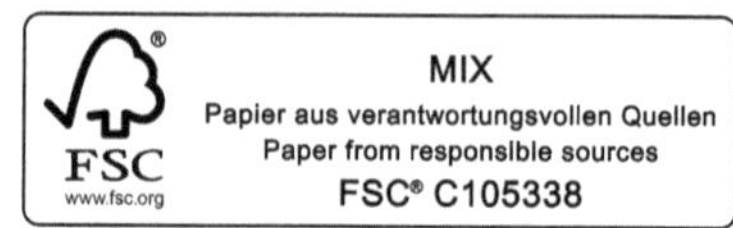

Printed by Books on Demand GmbH, Norderstedt / Germany